Published by Win-win Health Intellingence Limited
Food for Life copyright @ Win-win Health Intelligence Limited, 2022

All rights reserved. Without limiting the rights under copyright reserved above, no part of this publication may be reproduced, stored in or introduced into a database and retrieval system or transmitted in any form or any means (electronic, mechanical, photocopying, recording or otherwise) whitout the prior written permission of both the owner of the copyright and the above publishers.

First published 2022

Sold in aid of Yes to Life
UK Registered Charity 1112812

Acknowledgements

I owe an enormous debt of gratitude to everyone who has contributed to this book. In an extraordinary flood of generosity, we have had many recepies donated to make this wonderful project a reality.

By buying this book you will be supporting the work of Yes to Life.

Miquel Leon-Canete
Executive Director
Yes to Life

This book is dedicated
to everyone who makes our journey an enjoyable one.

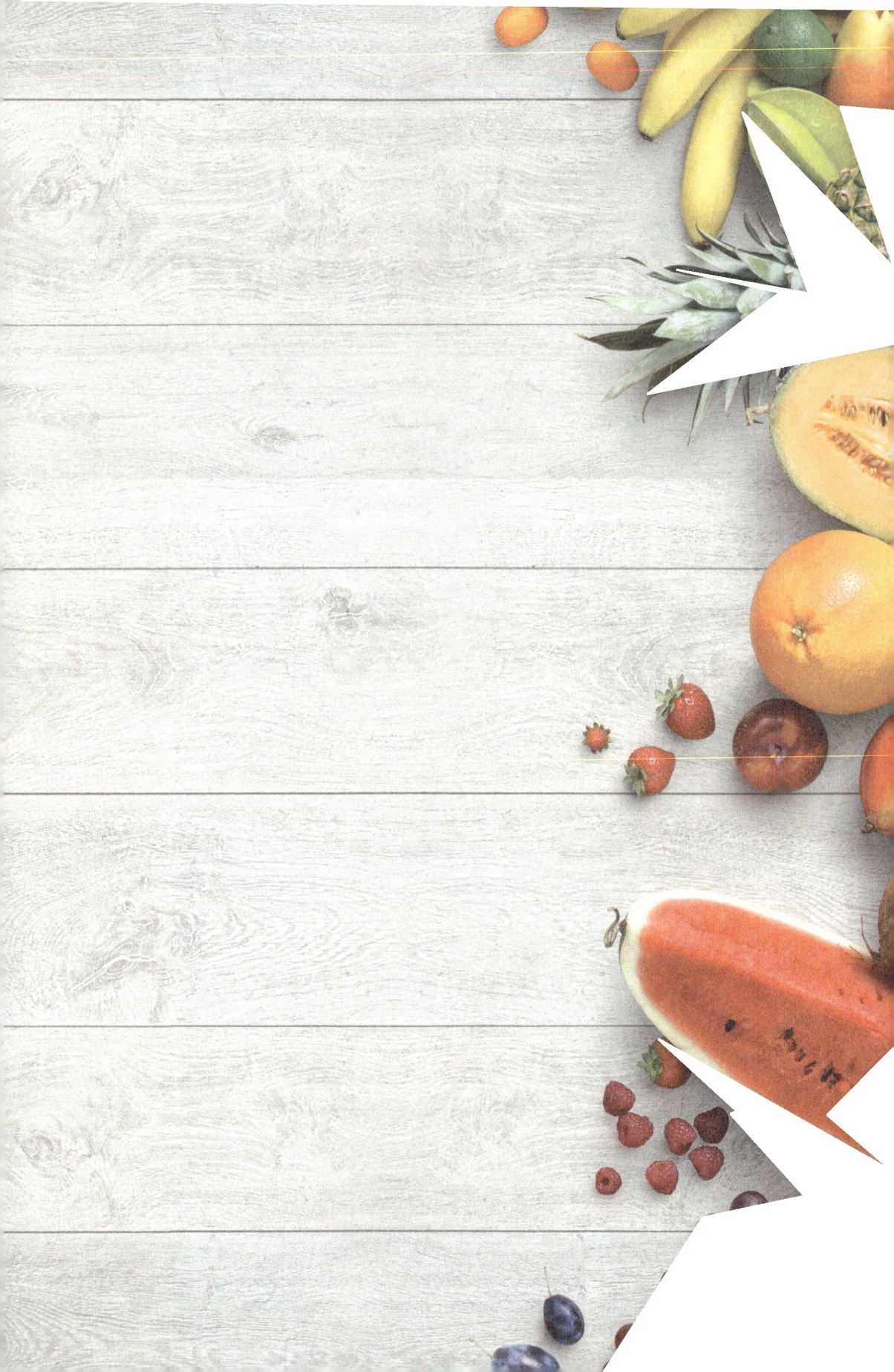

TABLE OF CONTENTS

01 Foreword by Kirsten Chick

03 Introduction by Robin Daly

05 Breakfast

17 Snacks

29 Salads and Sides

47 Mains

65 Desserts

75 Bread

82 Recipes Index

85 About Yes to Life

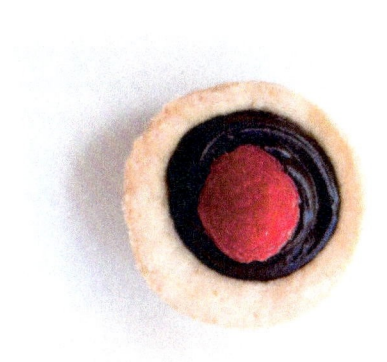

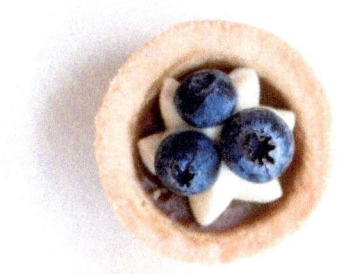

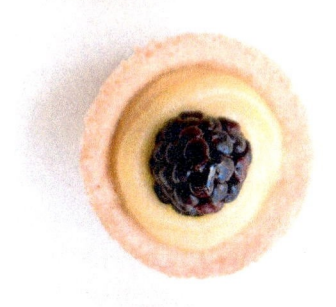

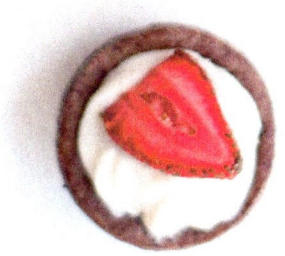

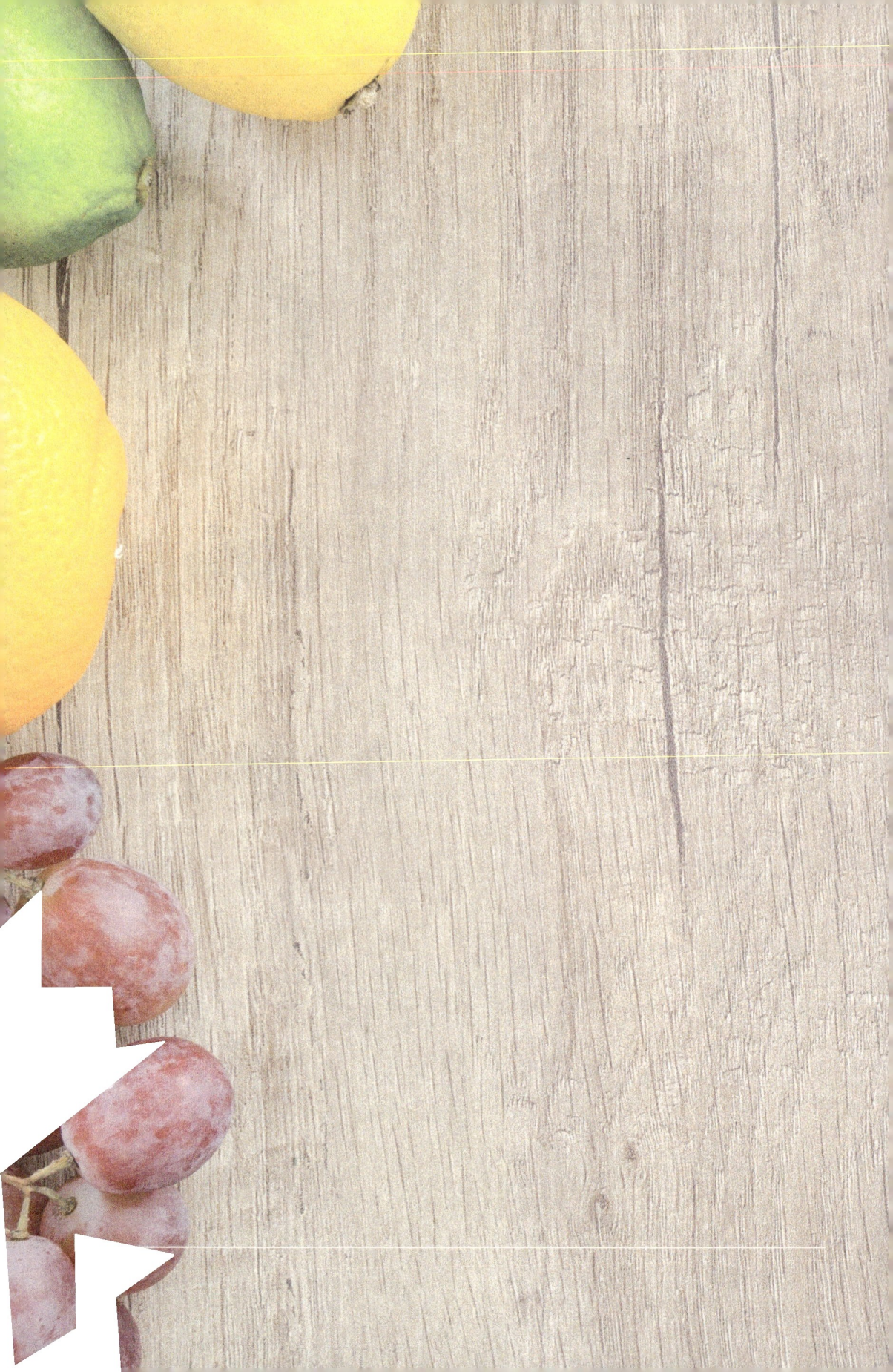

FOREWORD

Kirsten Chick
Nutritional therapist, nutrition educator, author and speaker.

Yes to Life is always there with practical support, a non-judgemental ear, a wealth of information and resources, an impressive network of professionals – and now this most wonderful, colourful, nourishing cook book, Food for Life.

It's rare that I am this excited about a collection of recipes. Most cookery books, however beautiful they look, really only offer a sprinkling of recipes I'll actually get round to trying. With Food for Life, however, I want to cook them all. They tick all my favourite boxes:

Vibrant – food that looks joyful is often more of a pleasure to eat, plus all those different colours represent a rainbow of anti-inflammatory, antioxidant and generally protective nutrients

Mouthwatering – if it's having this effect, then it's likely triggering all your digestive processes, so you'll be more deeply nourished by it

Balanced – helping you towards a supportive ratio of proteins, carbohydrates, fats/oils and fibre, that you can tweak for your own needs

Adaptable – many ingredients can be easily switched if there's one you don't eat

Inspiring – they make me want to try them out, play with variations and explore new ideas I haven't thought of before

Simple – I love my kitchen but don't want to spend all my time in there

As a nutritional therapist, I know how many of you will welcome this kind of inspiration and variety of ideas. I also know how important it is to feel excited by food, and to feel like there are a wealth of textures, tastes and colours open to you - whether you are living with, recovering from or seeking to prevent a cancer diagnosis.

Thankfully Food for Life is here to help blow away the myth that a healthy diet is bland and restrictive, and brighten up your mealtimes instead.

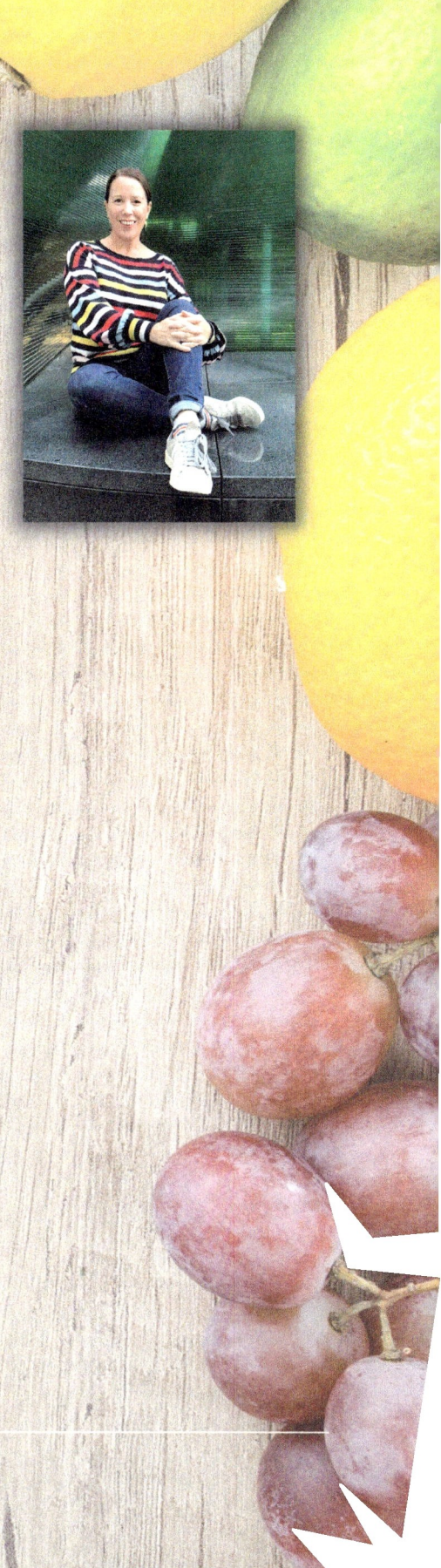

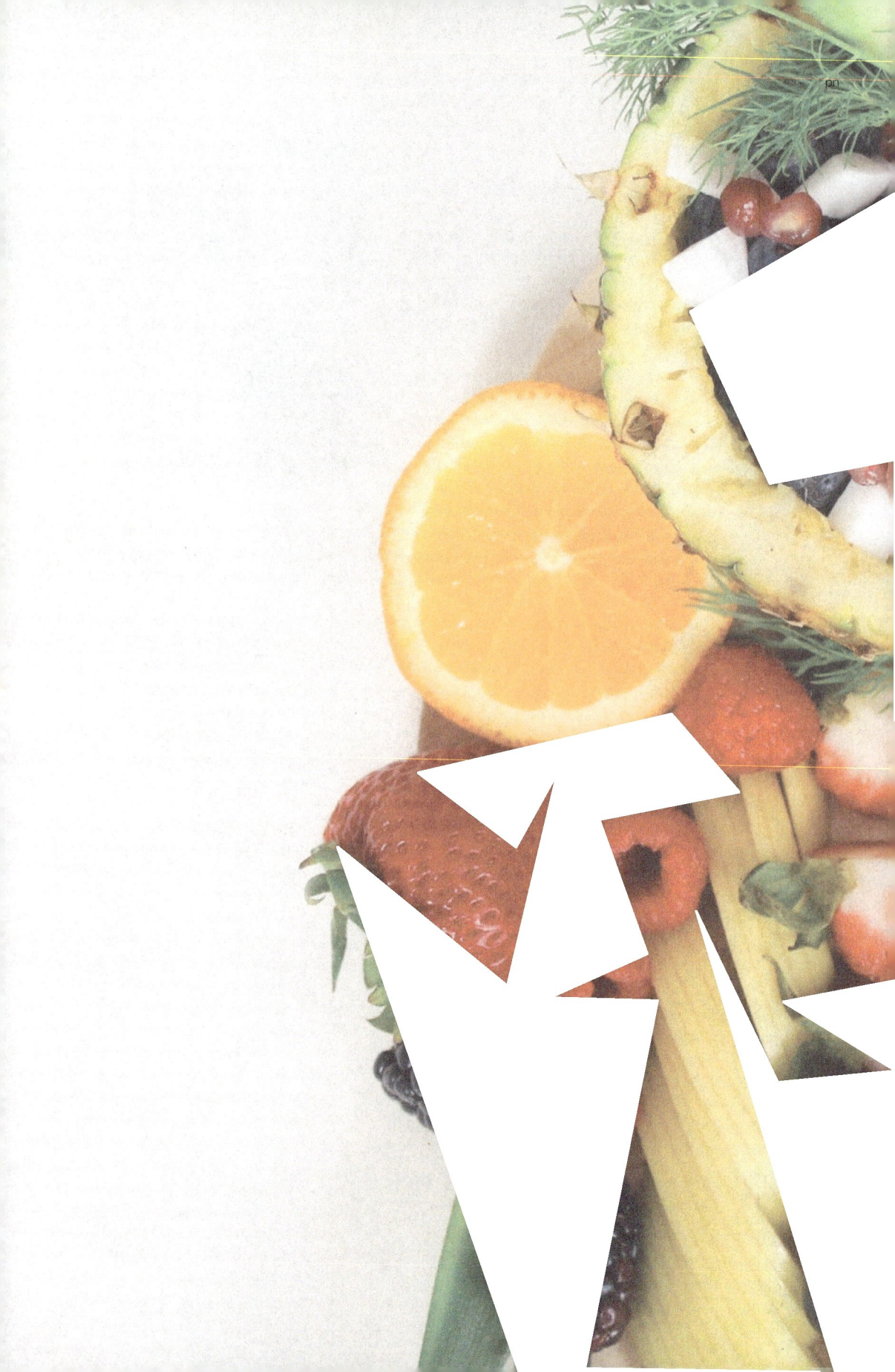

INTRODUCTION

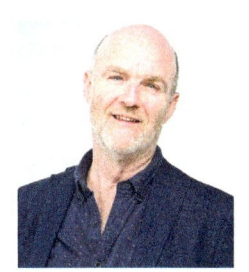

Robin Daly
Yes to Life Founder and Chair of Trustees

I'm immensely pleased and proud to be writing this introduction to our ravishing cookbook, Food for Life. This is not the first time in the last 18 years that we have made plans for a recipe book. Always we set out with the intention of collecting together tempting and delicious recipes, all under the watchful eye of a specialist Nutritional Therapist who could focus in on the value of the ingredients to those with cancer, both from the standpoint of the their therapeutic effects and the science behind them. It was simply an obvious lifestyle resource for Yes to Life to produce.

One way and another these plans never came to fruition... until now, that is! We have our energetic and dedicated Executive Director, Miquel Leon-Canete, to thank for finally making all the dreams into a reality, and with such style.

The first question anyone with a diagnosis of cancer who is starting to look for ways to help themselves will ask is 'What should I eat?' For far too long, this question has been dismissed as trivial and irrelevant by cancer specialists, but now the crucial importance of factors such as the health of the gut microbiome to treatment outcomes are a hot topic of mainstream research, and it's long past time to be underestimating the power of good nutrition to underpin the recovery of good health. Nutritional Therapist and long-term survivor of cancer Kirsten Chick needs little convincing of this, and her invaluable insights into, and overview of this project have played a key part in making the book such an irresistible go-to resource. Food for Life is a reflection of her broad view of nutrition, which encompasses the experiential, social, psychological and spiritual dimensions of eating – quite apart from the physical benefits to our biochemistry.

My sincere thanks go to all the many contributors who have enthusiastically and freely shared their culinary creativity and helped to make this book such an exceptional resource.

I hope you find great pleasure in exploring these pages. What more enjoyable way could there be to support your journey back to health than with such mouth-watering nourishment?

Robin Daly

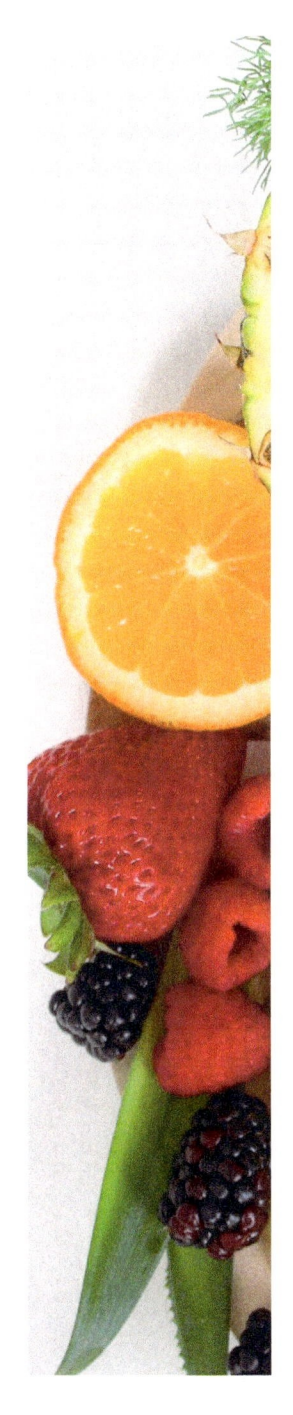

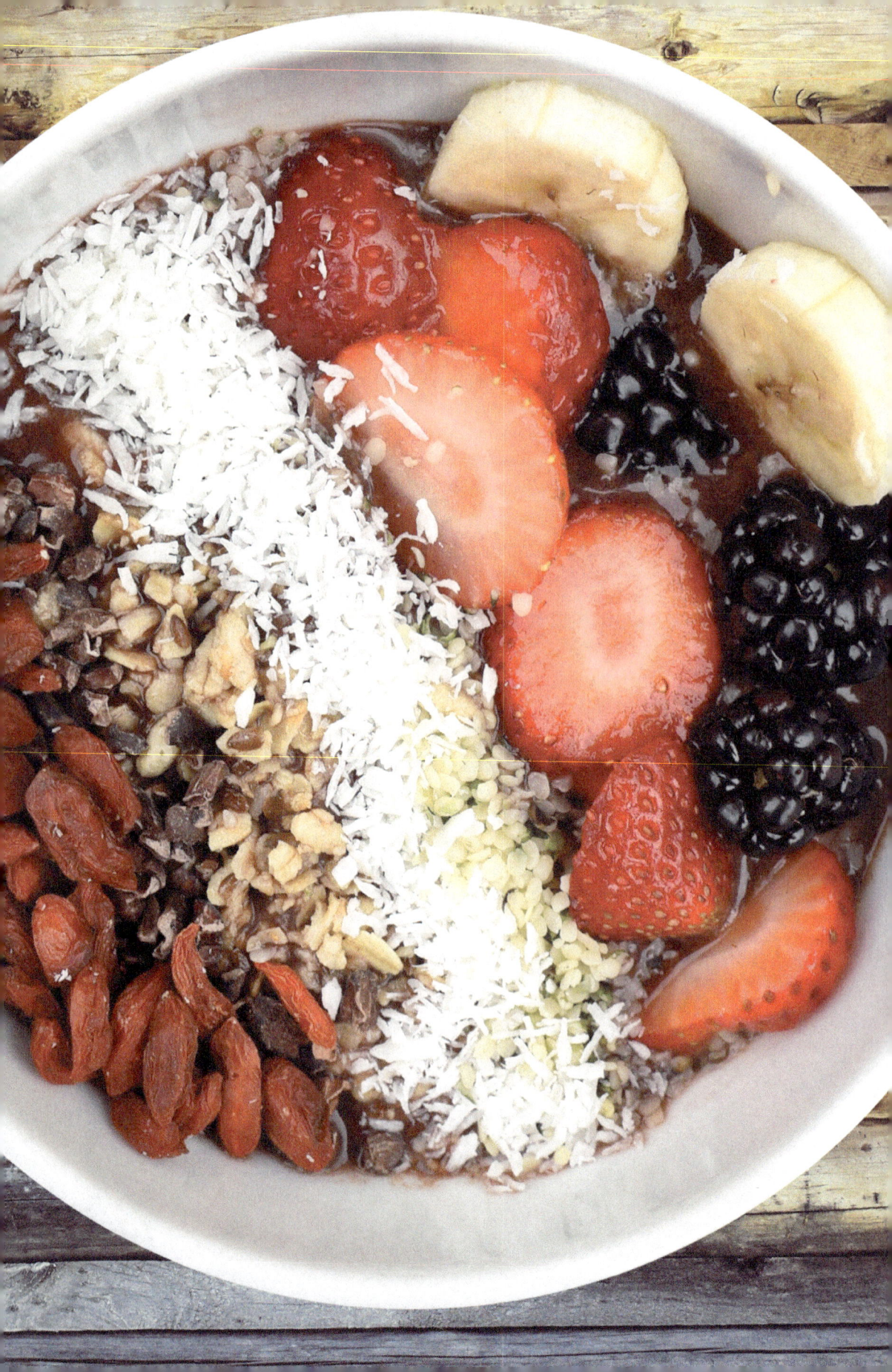

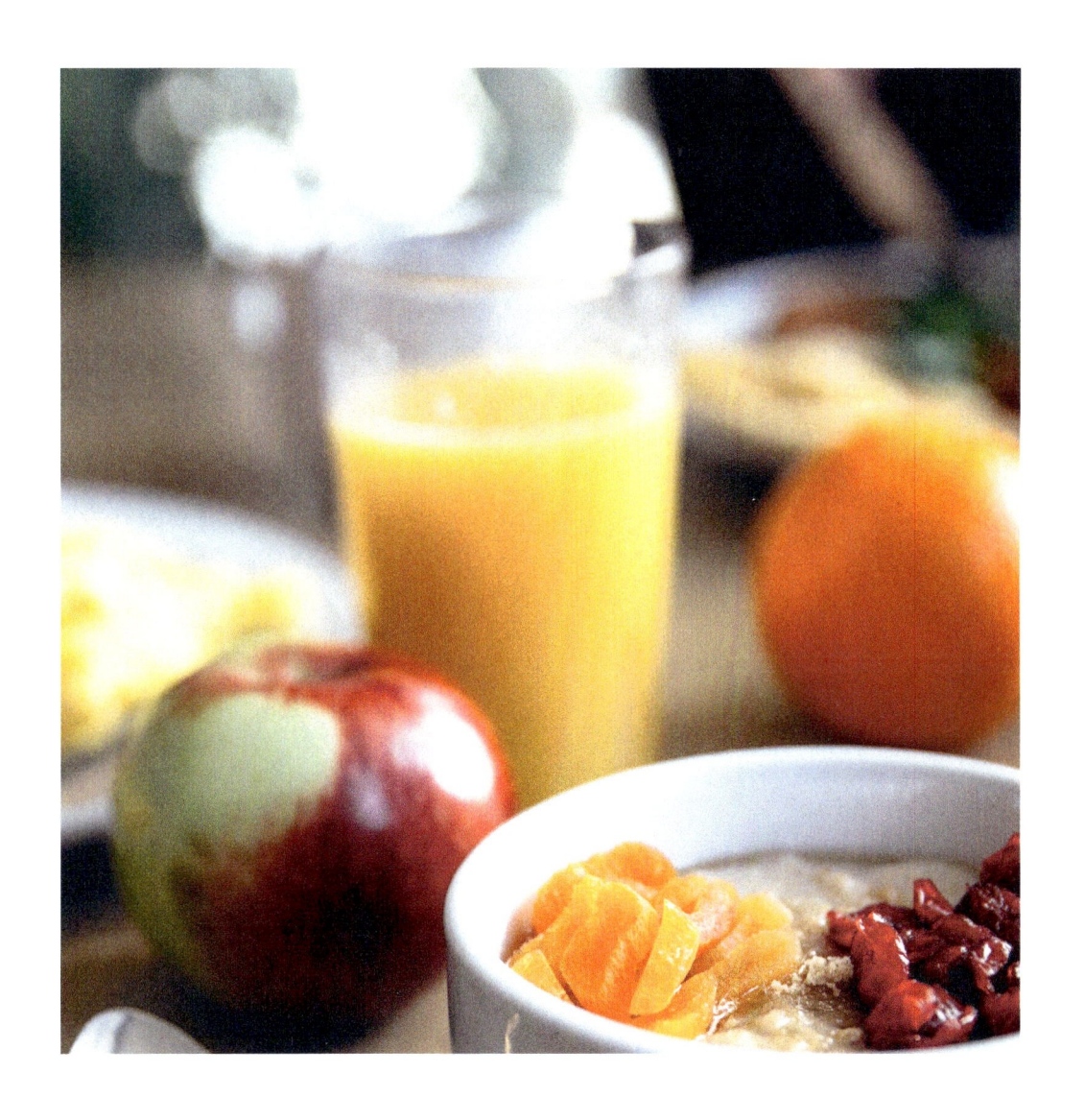

BREAKFAST

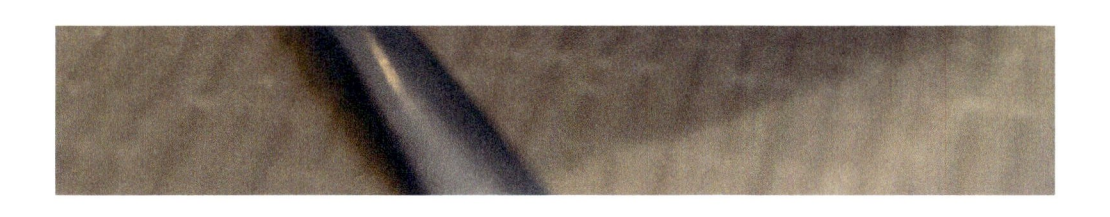

TROPICAL BIRCHER MUESLI

A dairy-free and gluten-free version of Bircher Muesli with a tropical twist — contains antioxidants, Omega 3, and fibre. Prepare the night before, for a hassle-free start to the day.

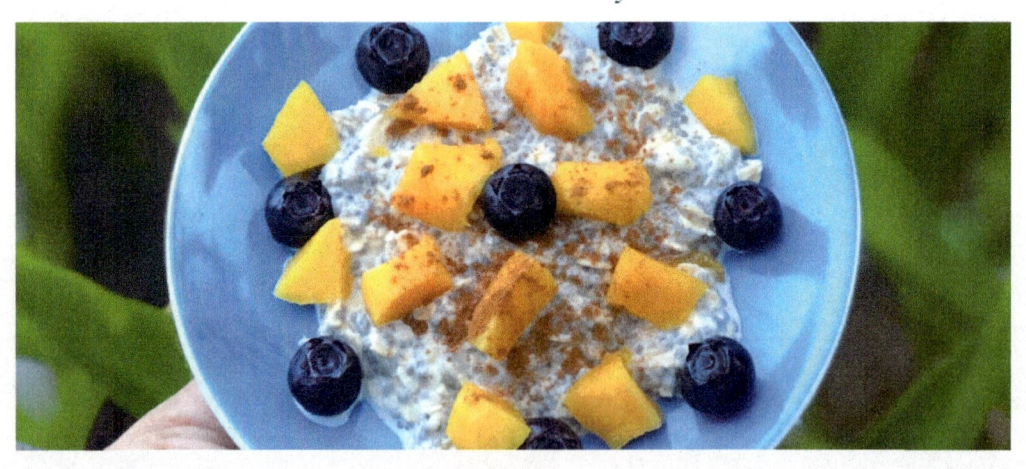

Ingredients

- 1 tbsp. chia seeds
- 3 tbsp. rolled oats (GF)
- ¼ cup sugar-free plant milk (cashew, almond, hazelnut, or oat)
- 1/2 mango
- 10-12 blueberries
- cinnamon powder
- chopped nuts (almonds, hazelnuts, etc.) and/or seeds (flax, chia, etc.)

Directions

1. Soak 1 tablespoon chia seeds and 3 tablespoons rolled oats (GF) in a ¼ cup plant milk (cashew, almond, hazelnut, coconut or oat) for at least 20 minutes and up to overnight.

2. Top with 1/2 a ripe cubed mango and 10-12 blueberries. Sprinkle with cinnamon powder.

3. Add a tablespoon of chopped nuts (almonds, hazelnuts, etc.) and/or seeds (flax, chia, etc.) for some protein and crunchiness.

4. Prepare a big portion and keep in the fridge for about 3 days; can also be enjoyed as a snack in the afternoon..

Recipe contributed by: The Cancer Coach, www.thecancercoach.org

OMELETTE FOR MUSHROOM LOVERS

Full of antioxidants and vitamin B this omelette is the perfect start to a busy day.

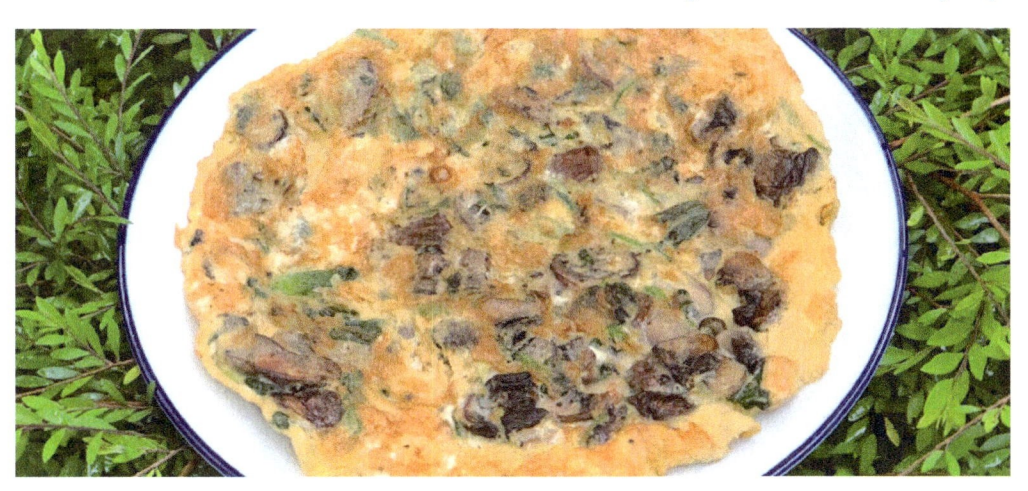

Ingredients

- 6 eggs (organic)
- 6 mushrooms
- 1 medium yellow onion
- 4 garlic cloves
- 3 spring onions
- 5 small tomatoes
- fresh basil leaves

Directions

1. Dice 6 mushrooms.
2. Chop 1 medium yellow onion.
3. Mince 4 garlic cloves.
4. Slice 3 spring onions, white and green parts.
5. Chop 5 small tomatoes.
6. Chop 5 fresh basil leaves.
7. Heat up a little bit of oil (extra virgin olive oil, extra virgin coconut oil or avocado oil) in a pan and fry all the ingredients until slightly brown.
8. Add the beaten egg, salt and pepper to taste. Continue cooking until your preferred consistency.

Recipe contributed by: The Cancer Coach, www.thecancercoach.org

TOO GOOD TO BE TRUE PANCAKES

You won't believe that these are gluten-free, dairy-free and have no added sugar. Ideal for a Sunday brunch treat for the whole family.

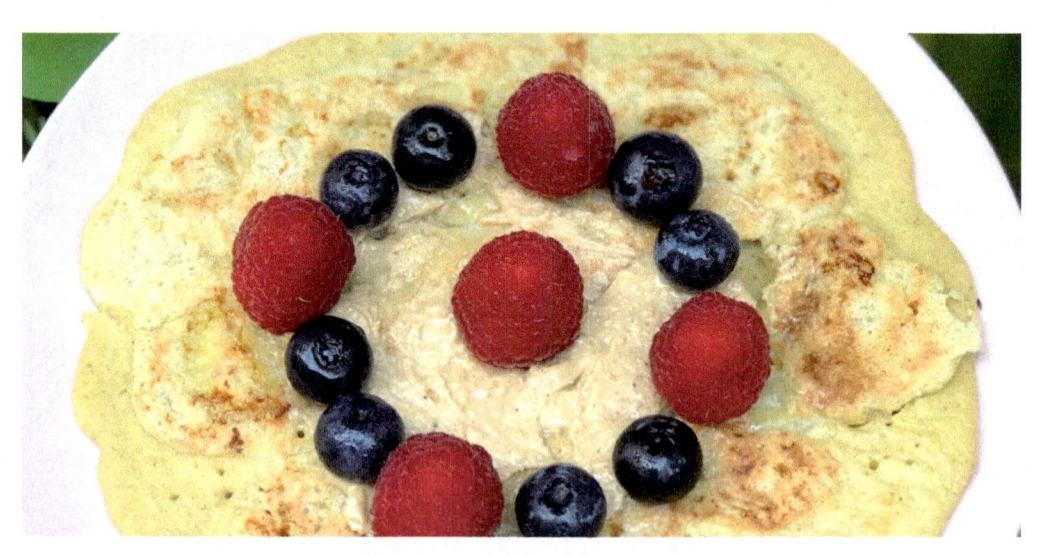

Ingredients

- 2 cups of organic oat flour (GF)
- 1 cup of almond milk or coconut milk
- 2 eggs
- 1 tsp. honey
- 1 tbsp. (spoon) avocado oil or coconut oil
- 1 pinch of salt
- For banana lovers: add 1 mashed banana or slices of banana

Directions

1. Stir everything together until the batter is just combined.

2. Don't over mix. Pour about ½ cup of batter into a non-stick or cast iron pan. You don't need to add any fat or oil to the pan.

3. Cook on low fire until bubbles appear, flip once and cook until set and light brown. Repeat with remaining batter until finished.

Note: These make thinner European-style pancakes that are a little thicker than a crepe.

Top with any of these
- *1 teaspoon good quality honey*
- *1 teaspoon of nut butter*
- *fresh fruits, like berries.*
- *sprinkle of cinnamon powder*

Recipe contributed by : Anonymous sender

FRUITY CHIA PORRIDGE

Enjoy your yummy breakfast!

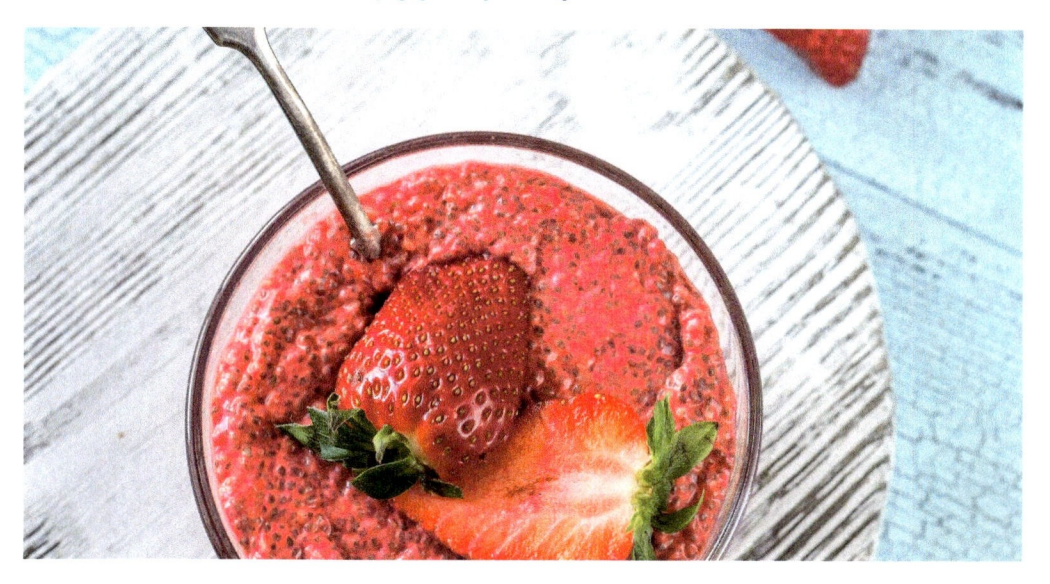

Ingredients

- 1-cup almond or coconut milk
- 1 tbsp. cashew or almond butter
- 1 tbsp. maple syrup or honey (optional)
- ½ cup chia seeds
- ¼ tsp. cinnamon
- 1 tsp. cacao nibs
- 1 tbsp. hemp seeds
- Handful blueberries
- Handful strawberries, chopped
- 1 banana, chopped

Directions

1. Pour the milk, cinnamon, maple syrup (if using sweetener) and nut butter into a blender or food processor and whizz for a minute
2. Pour into a bowl and add the chia seeds
3. Mix thoroughly and place in the fridge for about an hour (or prepare the night before)
4. Remove from fridge, add the fruits, hemp seeds and cacao nibs

Recipe contributed by : Anonymous sender

CHIA PUDDING

Prepare it in the evening for breakfast, or a mid-morning pick-me-up!

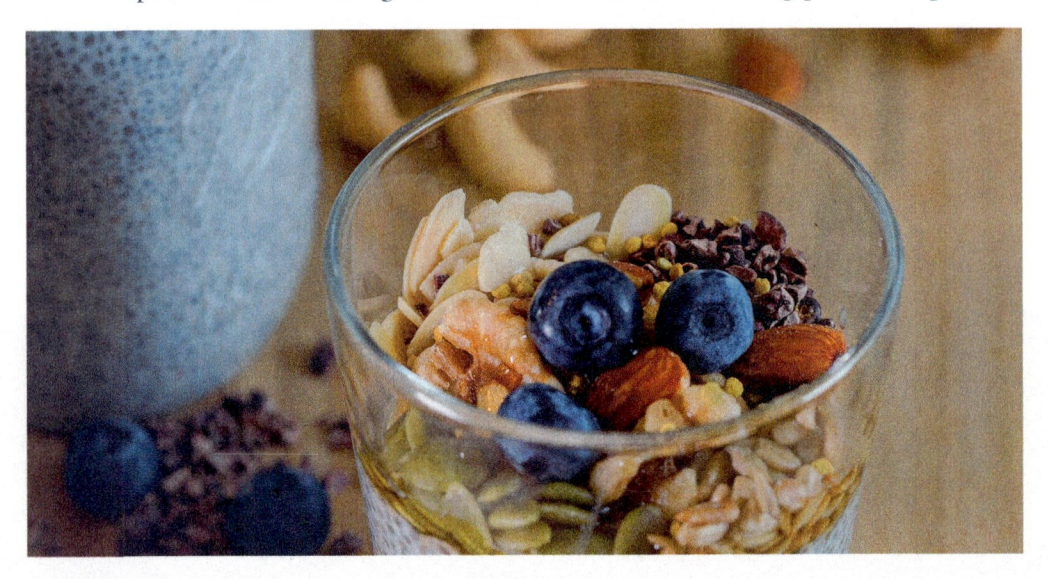

Ingredients

- 1/3 cup organic chia seeds
- 1 cup organic unsweetened almond milk
- 1 tsp. maple syrup (optional)
- 1/2 tsp. vanilla or cinnamon, to taste
- 1 glass jar with lid

Directions

1. Combine all the ingredients in a glass jar. Cover with lid and shake it few times

2. Wait for 5 minutes and shake it again

3. Refrigerate for at least 4 hours, or overnight

4. Chia seeds will expand and turn into a not too thick pudding

5. Top with berries, mango, or a sliced banana.... Sprinkle with nuts, unsweetened coconut flakes or cacao nibs.... or eat it like that!

You can add the unsweetened shredded coconut to the chia mix for a thicker consistency

Recipe contributed by: Silvia Mensurati, www.nutritiontoheal.com

CINNAMON SPICED SUPERSEED AND APRICOT CHEWY FLAPJACKS

These chewy, oaty flapjacks are made with gorgeously sweet apricots, bananas and maple syrup, and Cinnamon Spice Superseeds add the perfect amount of crunch.

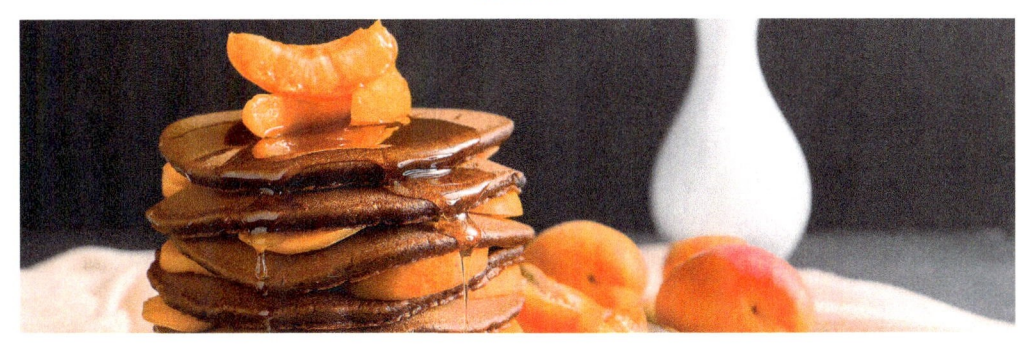

Ingredients

DRY

- 2 cups of oats (gluten free)
- 1 tsp. cinnamon
- ½ tsp mixed spice
- ½ cup Cinnamon Spice Superseeds
- ½ cup chopped apricots (chopped into pea-sized chunks)

WET

- 2 bananas mashed
- 5 tbsp maple syrup (or honey)
- ¼ cup rapeseed oil (or melted coconut oil)
- 1 tsp. vanilla extract

Recipe from Food for Life series, Yes to Life

Directions

1. Set the oven to 180°C. Line a 30cm square brownie tray.
2. Combine the dry ingredients and wet ingredients in two separate bowls.
3. Add the wet to the dry and mix well.
4. Pour mix into the brownie tray, ensuring the mix is packed evenly.
5. Bake for 25-30 minutes (Check after 20. If it is browning too much, cover loosely in foil).
6. Remove and let cool completely before slicing into squares.
7. Store in an airtight container for up to 5 days.

ZESTY FRESH SUMMER CHIA PUDDING

This is a recipe you make the night before. Overnight breakfasts are great for removing decision-making from your morning. So rather than being tempted by a sugary cereal you have it right there, ready for you

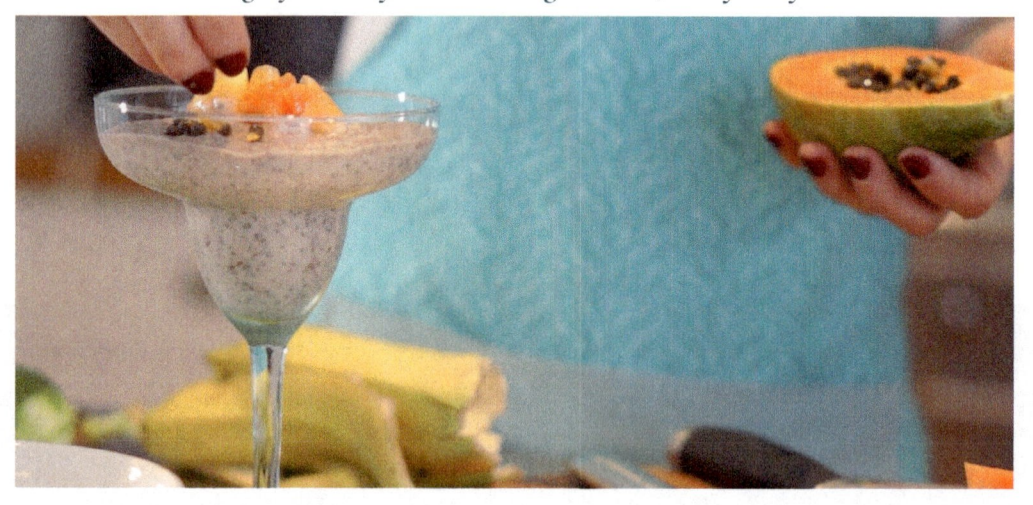

Ingredients

- The zest of 1/2 a lime
- 1/2 cup pitted, roughly chopped, soaked dates (soak for 10 minutes in warm water, drain but keep the water, it's great to add to a smoothie or to have as a pre-workout drink)
- 1/2 cup ground almonds, freshly ground or pre-ground
- 1 cup of water
- 2 tbsp. chia seeds

Toppings (optional)

- *Shaved papaya*
- *Papaya seeds*
- *Ground cacao nibs*

Directions

1. Blend all the pudding ingredients together, except the chia seeds, till smooth.
2. You can use a jug or hand blender for this.
3. Mix in the chia seeds and pour into bowls. Leave in the fridge overnight.
4. Add the toppings in the morning and eat!

Recipe from Food for Life series, Yes to Life

Although every ingredient in this recipe is a nutritional powerhouse, I will focus on the following:

Bananas: High in potassium, slow-release carbohydrates, great to start the morning with

Chia seeds: Source of protein, for 100g you have 34% of your RDA, high in fibre which is awesome in the morning to get the bowel moving. High in Omega Fatty Acids (essential fatty acids, Omega 3) which help raise HDL (good cholesterol) and reduce LDL (bad cholesterol). Also rich in iron and calcium

Papaya seeds: Not many know this, but Papaya seeds are pretty much nutritional medicine! They contain nutrients that help cleanse the liver and kidneys (cleansing). Even patients with cirrhosis of the liver benefit from the compounds and anti-oxidants in this wonderful seed. It is anti-inflammatory and helps with arthritis and joint pain! But mostly, it is awesome for the gut with seeds being a great remedy for killing intestinal parasites!

Food tips
- *This is a breakfast you make the night before. Overnight breakfasts are great for removing decision-making from your morning. So rather than being tempted by a sugary cereal you have it right there, ready for you.*
- *You can make this in sealed container and take it with you for a breakfast to eat on your commute or at work*
- *Great for kids as it's like dessert but much healthier than most cereals*

BROCCOLI GUACAMOLE WITH POACHED EGG

A delicious breakfast for guacamole lovers.

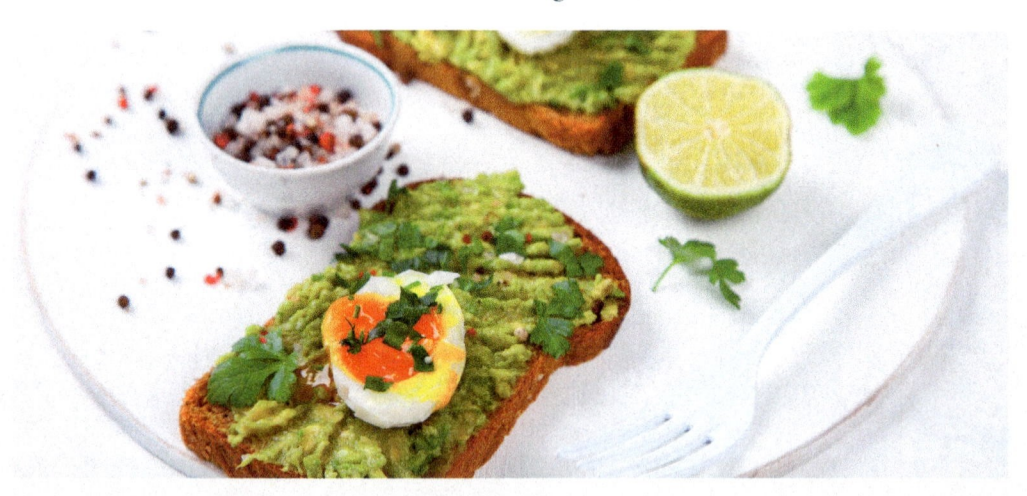

Ingredients

- 2 eggs
- 4 sundried tomatoes
- 4 broccoli florets, cooked
- 2 tbsp. soft goats cheese, or olive oil if you are dairy free
- 1 avocado
- Salt and pepper
- Flax or rye bread

Directions

1. Poach the eggs. You can use an electric steamer – adding the eggs to a silicon poach pod and steaming for 8-10 minutes.
2. Add the broccoli, avocado and goat's cheese or oil to a small blender and whizz until smooth.
3. Check the consistency and add a dash of hot water if required. Give a final whizz.
4. Spread the guacamole over a slice of flax or rye bread and top with the sundried tomatoes.
5. Loosen the egg in the pod by running a knife around the outside.
6. Cut a criss cross pattern and pop out over the tomatoes.

Recipe contributed by: Jenny Phillips, www.inspirednutrition.co.uk

A TASTE OF TUSCANY ON TOAST

Tuscany is one of my favorite spots in the world. This popular, simple and rustic Italian dish takes me there.

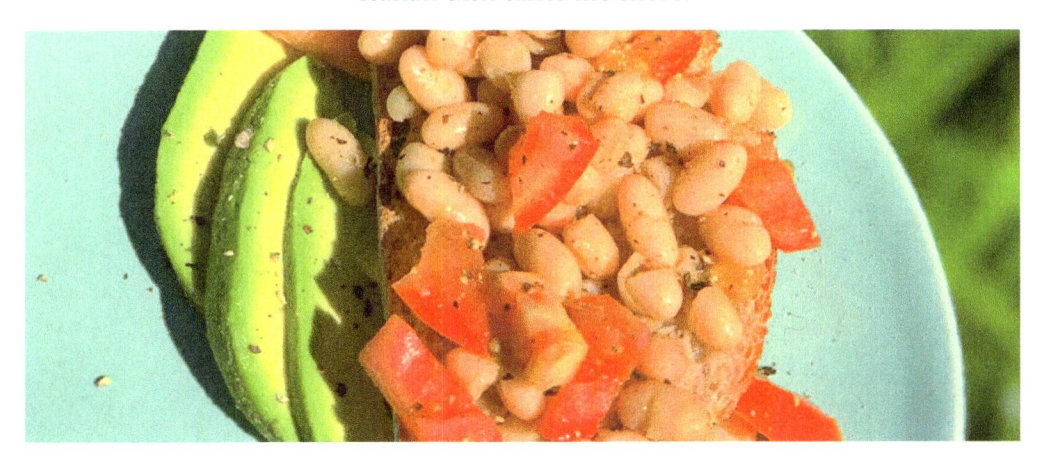

Ingredients

- Cannellini beans (or white kidney beans)
- One cubed tomato
- One avocado
- Extra virgin olive oil

Directions

1. Mix the boiled cannellini beans* with one cubed tomato, drizzle with extra virgin olive oil, add fresh or dried oregano, salt and pepper to taste.

2. Add this delicious combination of flavor to rustic sourdough toast (GF).

3. Add a few slices of avocado on the side for creamy goodness that pairs well with the beans.

*I usually avoid using canned food, but I do like to have some canned organic beans in my pantry for busy mornings or for a quick side dish when time is short.

Cannellini beans (or white kidney beans) are nutritious—high in protein (1/4 cup serving contains 11 grams of protein), an excellent source of fibre, folate, iron and magnesium. They also contain a wealth of B vitamins, including B12.

Recipe contributed by: The Cancer Coach, www.thecancercoach.org

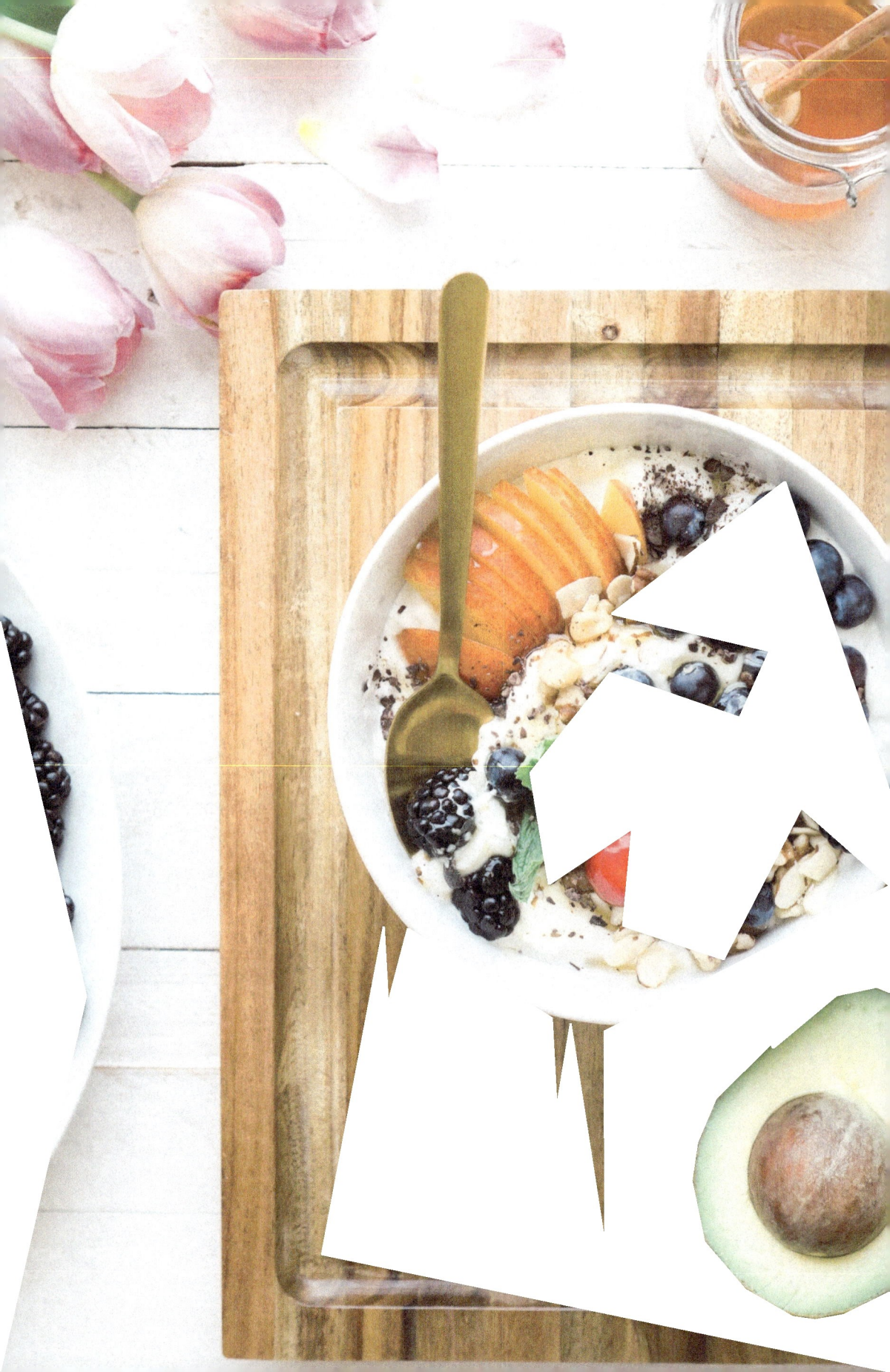

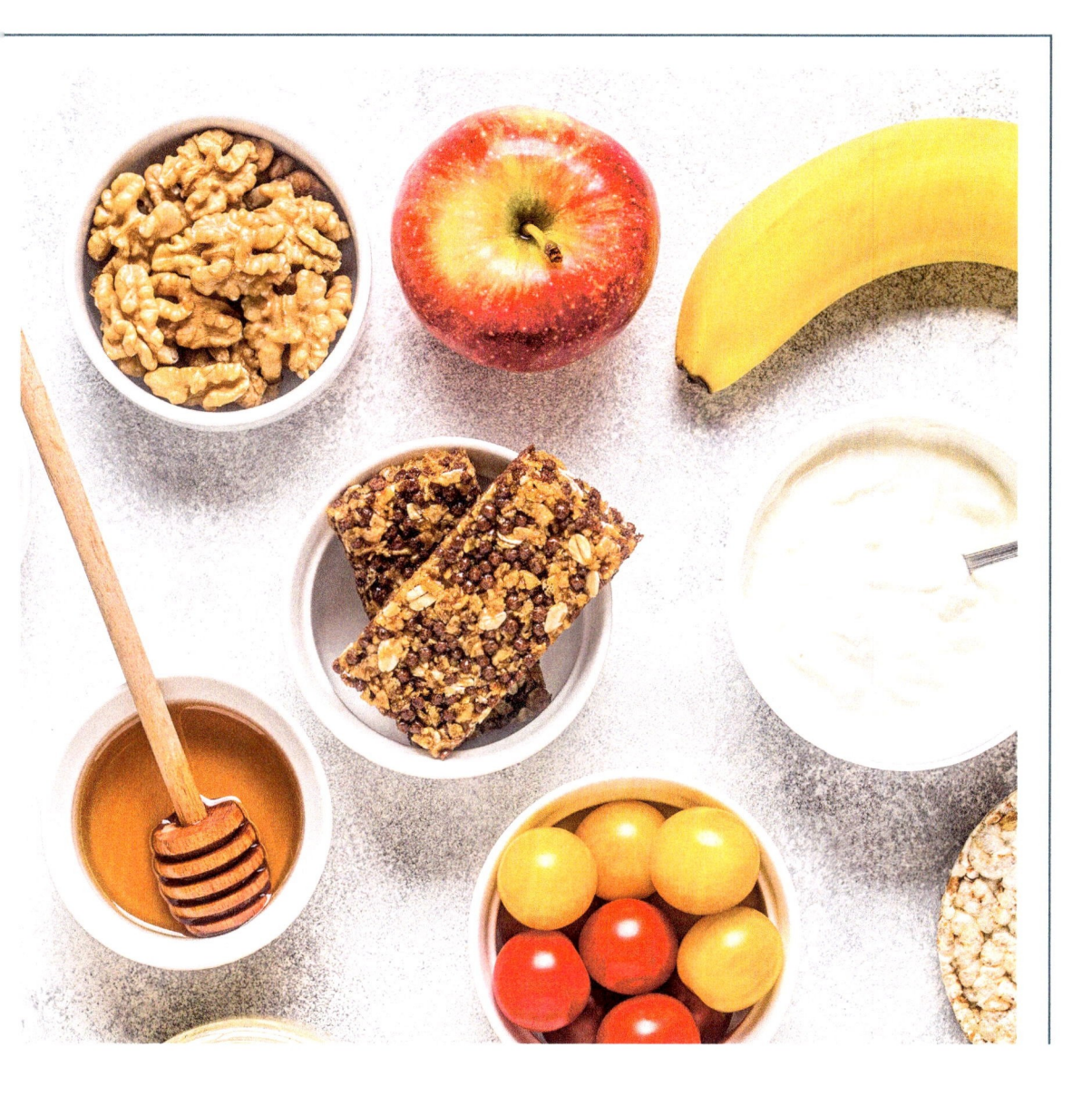

SNACKS

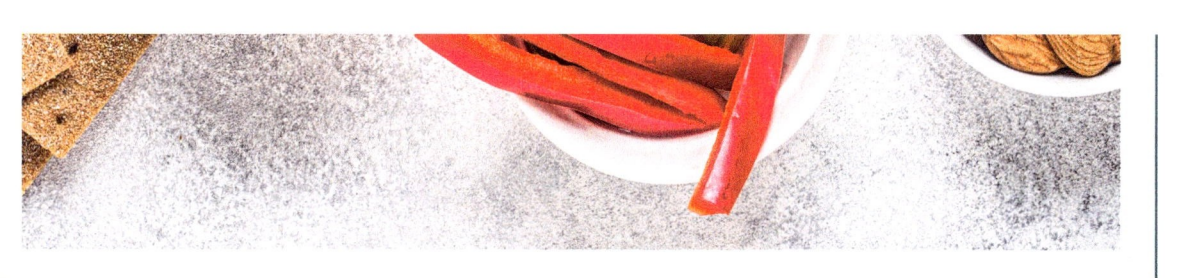

CHIA FRESH SUMMER SMOOTHIE

All you need to get the Chia power.

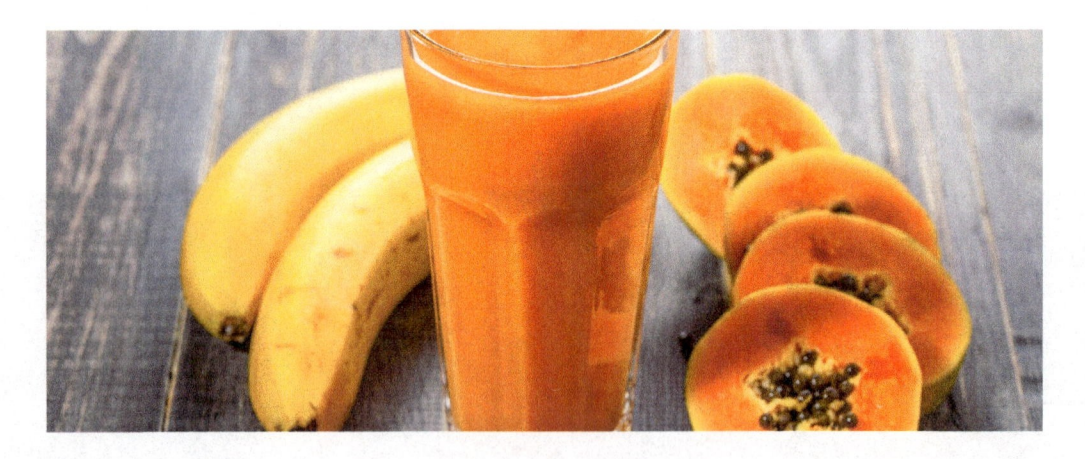

Ingredients

- 4 medium bananas
- ½ cup of dates (pitted, roughly chopped and soaked for 10 minutes in hot water)
- ½ cup of ground almonds
- 1 cup of water
- The zest of ½ a lime
- 2 tbsp. chia seeds
- Toppings (optional): Shaved papaya, papaya seeds, ground cacao nibs

Directions

1. Blend all the pudding ingredients together, except the chia seeds, till smooth.

2. You can use a jug or hand blender for this.

3. Mix in the chia seeds and pour into bowls.

4. Leave in the fridge overnight.

5. Add the toppings in the morning and eat!

Recipe from Food for Life series, Yes to Life

BEAUTIFUL BEETROOT DIP

Expect the unexpected with these flavours.

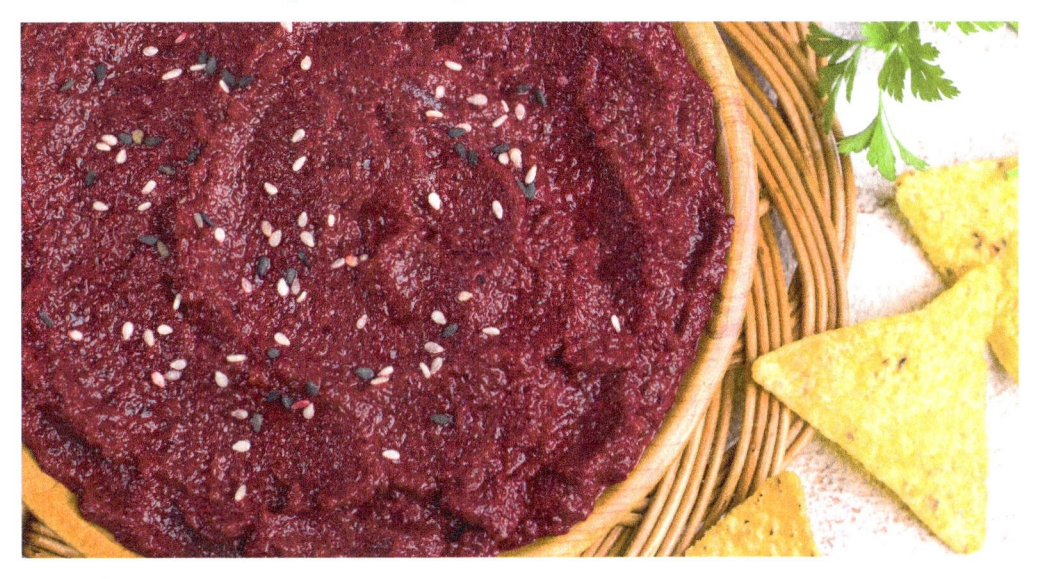

Ingredients

- 2 medium sized beetroots, peeled and chopped
- 1 medium red onion, peeled and chopped
- 1 clove of garlic, peeled
- 35g sunflower seeds
- 2 tbsp. olive oil
- 2 tbsp. tahini
- Juice of half a lemon

Directions

1. Place all the ingredients in a food processor.
2. Switch on and mix until the ingredients are well blended.
3. Store in a glass jar for up to 3 days and use generously

Recipe contributed by: Jenny Phillips, www.inspirednutrition.co.uk

CRUNCHY APPLE–CINNAMON SNACK

A delicious mid-morning or late-afternoon snack with a yummy flavour of apple pie that is nutrient dense and rich in antioxidants, fibre, and protein.

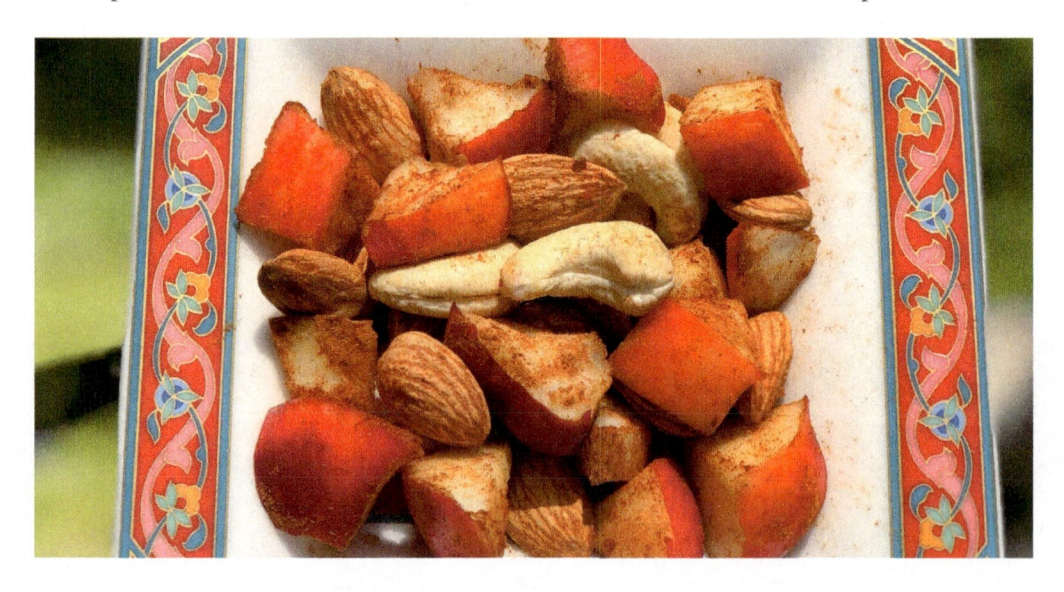

Ingredients

- 1/2 red apple
- Handful of nuts
- Handful of pumpkin seeds

Directions

1. Toss together in a bowl ½ of a red apple cut into cubes, a small handful of nuts (cashews, walnuts, or almonds) and a small handful of pumpkin seeds (pepitas).

2. Shake cinnamon powder over the top.

Recipe contributed by: The Cancer Coach, www.thecancercoach.org

MICROWAVE HUMMUS – FROM MINIMALIST BAKERS

Lovely warm, but keeps in fridge for a few days and thickens

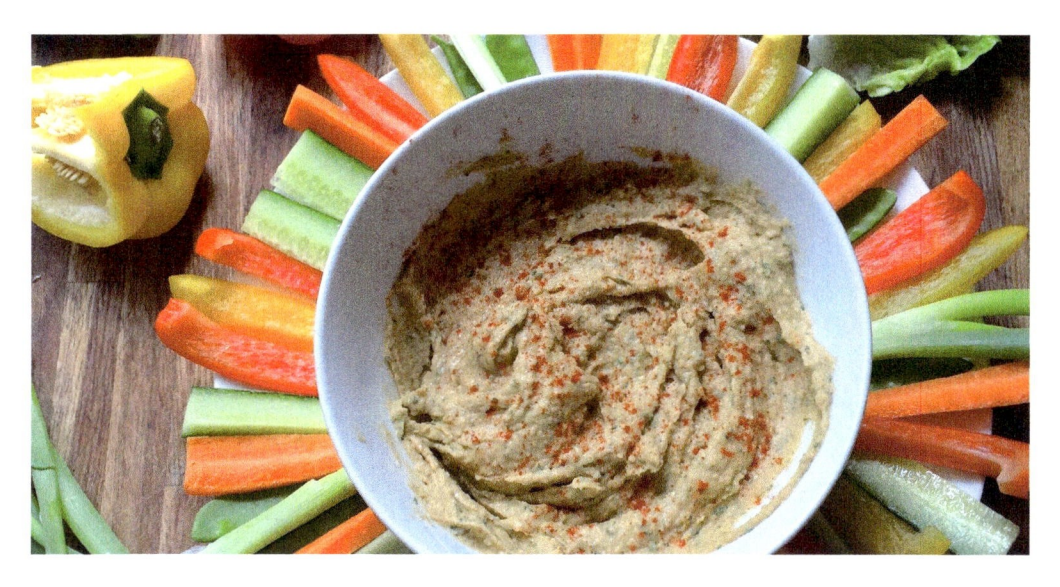

Ingredients

- Can of chick peas (in water)
- Peeled garlic cloves (4/5)
- Splash of olive oil
- Peanut butter to taste
- 1 lemon

Directions

1. Microwave for 4 mins.
2. Blitz in blender.
3. Add peanut butter, lemon juice, splash olive oil.

Optional: add spices like smoked paprika or cumin

You can add beetroot or peas or olives & sundried tomatoes for another flavour.

All yummy

Recipe contributed by: Karin Ayres

FLAX & PUMPKIN TURMERIC THINS

Crispy, nutritious, savoury flax seeds thins that will make you come back for more!

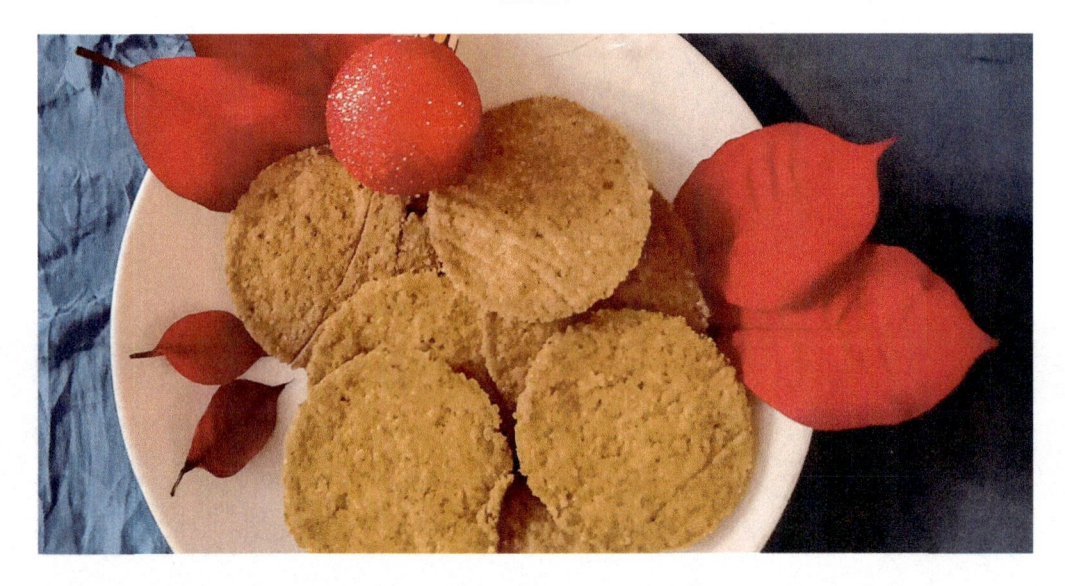

Ingredients

- 1 cup flax seeds
- 4 tbsp. pumpkin seeds
- ½ tsp. turmeric powder
- ¼ tsp. chilli flakes
- ½ tsp. good quality sea salt (optional)
- ½ cup water

Directions

1. Preheat the oven to 180C, 160 fan, gas mark 4.

2. Grind the flax and pumpkin seeds and add them to a medium-size bowl with the turmeric, chilli and salt, if using. Mix well.

3. Add the water and mix well.

4. With clean hands, form a dough and shape it into a ball.

5. If the dough is too sticky, add some more flax meal.

6. Place the ball between two pieces of parchment paper and, using a rolling pin, roll it to your desired thickness.

7. Cut the dough into circles with the help of a glass. Roll any extra into more thins.

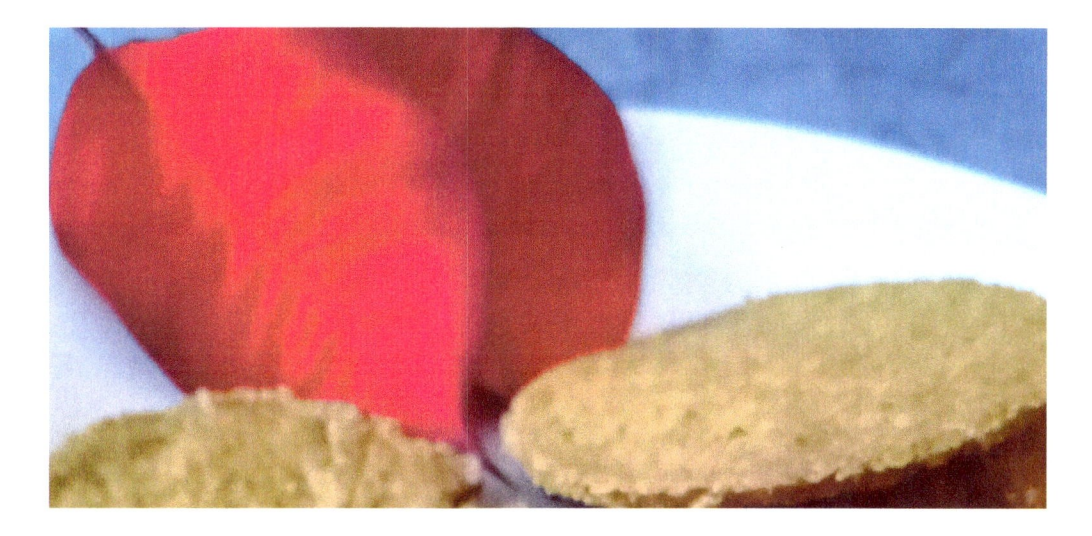

8. Remove the piece of parchment paper on top, and slide the paper with the thins on a baking sheet.

9. Prick each cracker with a fork.

10. Bake until golden. Baking time depends on the thickness of your thins, the thicker they are, the longer it will take to bake them.

11. I like my thins quite thin, so they are ready in 7 minutes or so.

12. Check them frequently to prevent burning.

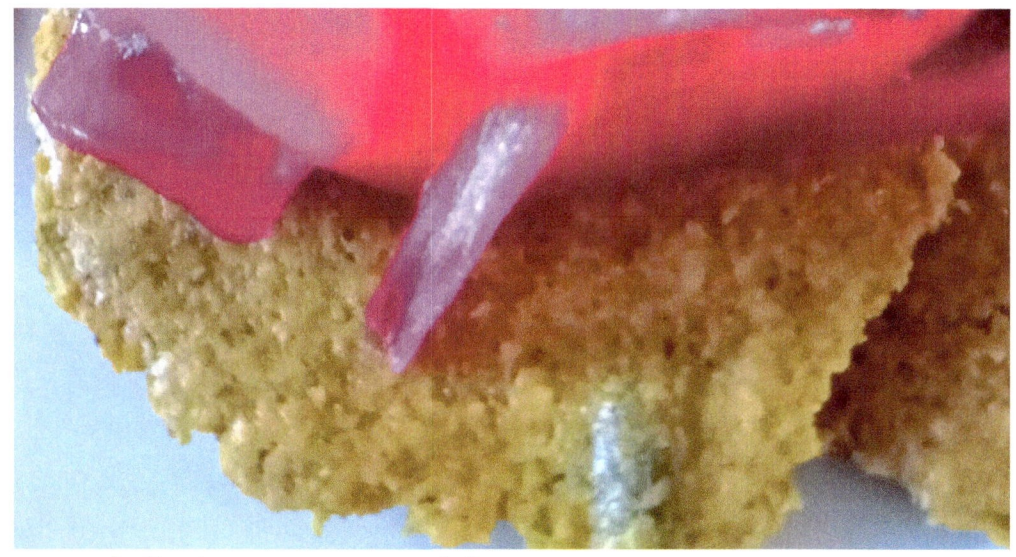

Recipe contributed by: Silvia Mensurati, www.nutritiontoheal.com

BUZZ-WORTHY SNACK

High in antioxidants and fibre, the creamy texture of the coconut yoghurt combined with the crunchiness of the bee pollen tastes divine. Bee pollen, a powerful immunity booster, is loaded with antioxidants and has anti-inflammatory and antimicrobial properties.

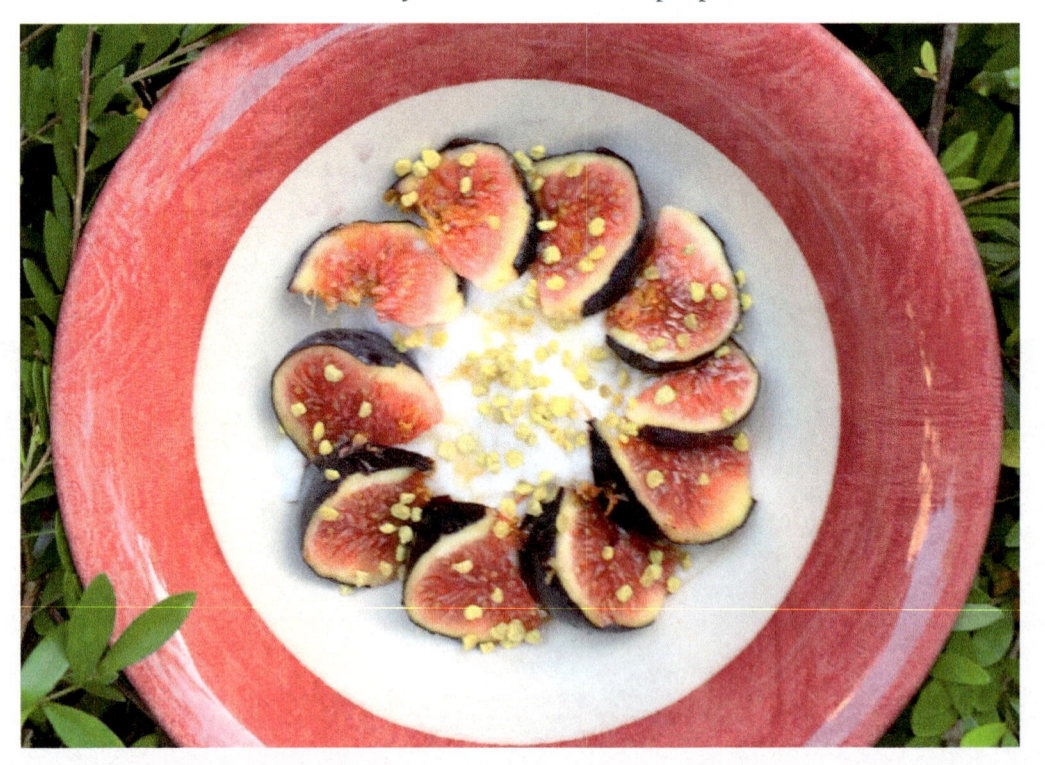

Ingredients

- 4 scoops of coconut yoghurt
- 1 fresh fig
- 1 tsp. of bee pollen

Directions

1. Put 4 scoops of coconut yoghurt (dairy free) into a bowl.
2. Top with one fresh fig cut into slices (you can also use other fruits, like berries or apple).
3. Sprinkle with 1 teaspoon of bee pollen.

Recipe contributed by: The Cancer Coach, www.thecancercoach.org

TAMARI SEEDS

These are the perfect snack for when you want something salty and crunchy, but want something more sustaining and wholesome than crisps.
They're also great as a salad topping or soup garnish, or to sprinkle on your porridge.

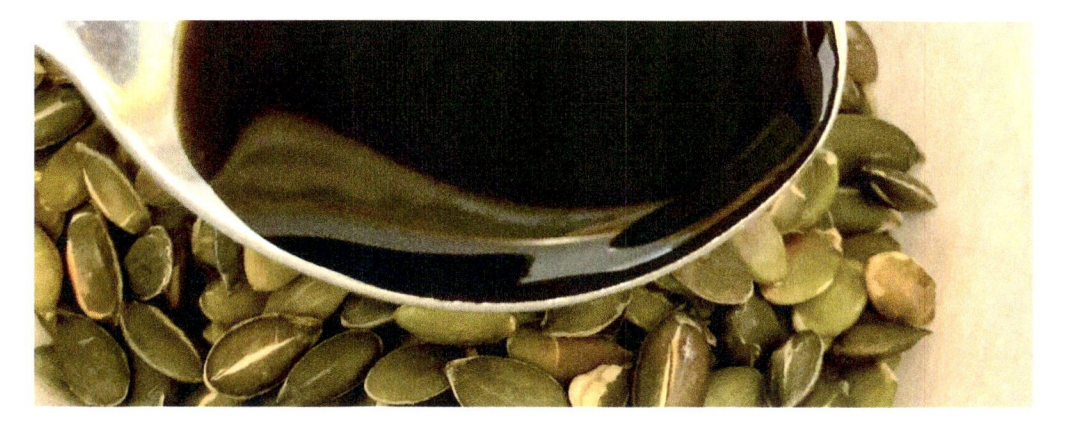

Ingredients

- 450-100g pumpkin seeds
- 1-2 tbsp. tamari (wheat-free soy sauce)

Directions

1. Add seeds to a dry frying pan (i.e. no oil or water), and heat over a gentle to moderate heat, shaking the pan from time to time.

2. After a few minutes, the seeds will start to pop – pour them into a bowl withini a minute or two of this, before they burn.

3. Sprinkle with tamari and quickly stir through.

4. Transfer to an airtight glass jar when cool and snack on as required.

Variations:
·Use sunflower seeds instead
·Use a mix of pumpkin, sunflower and sesame seeds – but add the pumpkin seeds first, then add the sunflower seeds, and then the sesame seeds, as they will all have different cooking times
·Stir in finely chopped (fresh or dried) herbs with the tamari
·Stir in ground paprika with the tamari
·Add dried chilli flakes and/or whole cumin seeds to the seeds as they cook

Recipe contributed by: Kirsten Chick (kirstenchick.com)

SUPER GREEN SMOOTHIE

Give yourself a morning or afternoon boost with a shake packed with antioxidants, omega 3 and protein. Chlorella is a protein-packed type of algae that is also rich in B12, iron, and vitamin C.

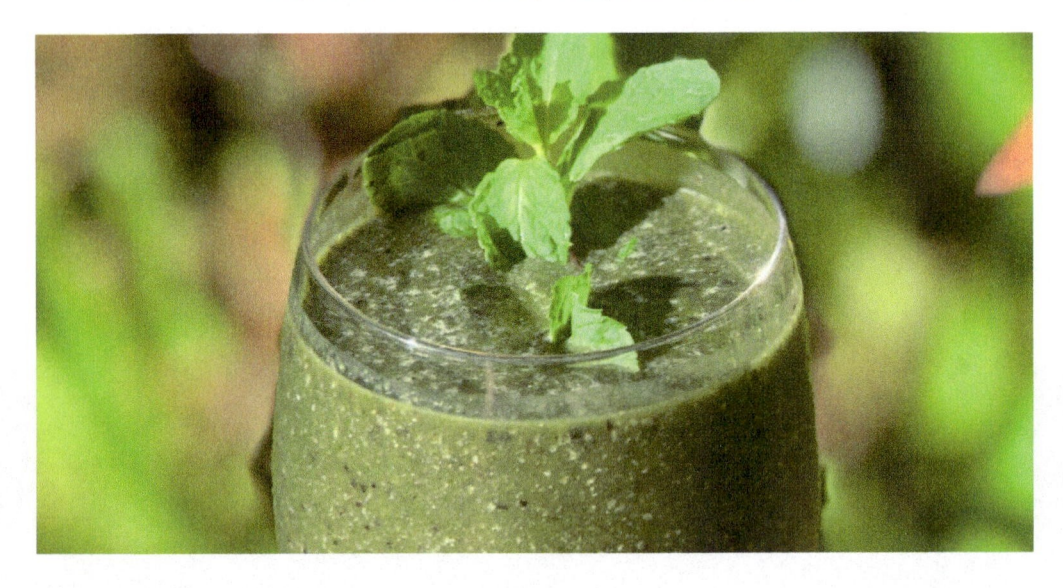

Ingredients

- 3/4 cup of nut milk (dairy free and sugar free) or 3/4 cup of coconut water
- 1 tbsp. chia seeds
- 1 big handful of raw young spinach leaves
- 10-12 fresh mint leaves
- 1/2 banana
- 1/2 cup of blueberries
- 1 tsp. of chlorella
- 1 tsp. protein powder (optional)

Directions

1. Mix all ingredients in a blender.
2. Add a little more or less liquid (water, nut milk or coconut water) to achieve your preferred consistency.

Recipe contributed by: The Cancer Coach, www.thecancercoach.org

HEALTHY VEGAN CRACKERS

When you fancy a crunch but you want something healthy,
try these vegan, paleo, gluten free crackers!
They're easy to make yet delicious and you'll wonder why
you never tried them before.

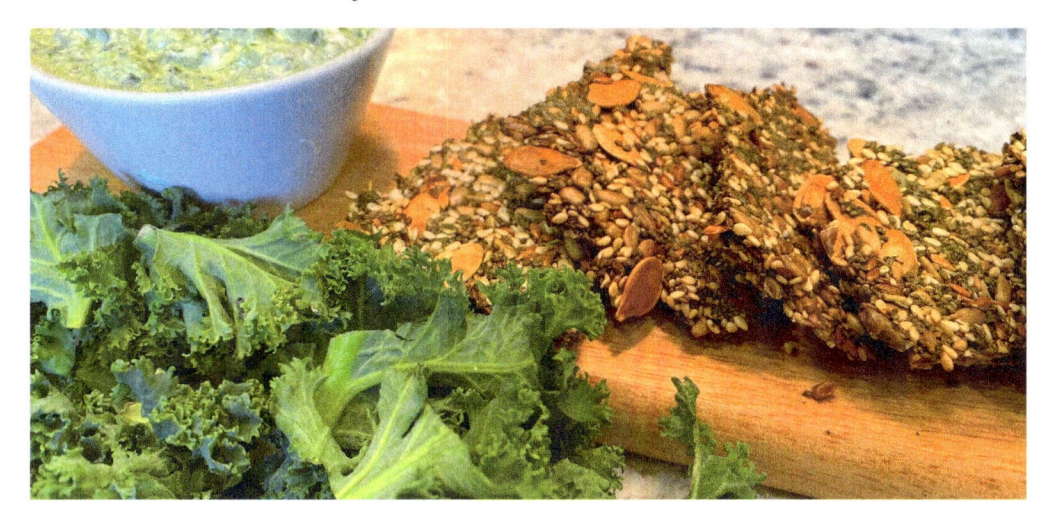

Ingredients

- 1 sachet Britt's superfoods organic kale juice
- Big handful of finely chopped kale
- 64g pumpkin seeds
- 32g chia seeds
- 64g sunflower seeds
- 1 tbsp. flaxseeds
- 1 tbsp. poppy seeds
- 1 tspb. sea salt
- 2 tsp. garlic salt
- 1 tsp. dried basil
- 6 oz water

Directions

1. You simply mix all the ingredients together and leave to stand for about 15 minutes. This is important as the seeds need to soak up the water.

2. Then transfer to a lined baking sheet and place another sheet of lined paper on top and roll the mixture until cracker thickness.

3. Cook at 180 degrees for about 25 minutes until the edges start to brown and then remove from oven and carefully cut into slices and turn before returning to the oven for five minutes to firm up.

4. We paired them with a wild garlic dip - and they didn't last for long!

"These crackers are healthy, simple and taste great, fantastic with a veggie spread or on their own. The only question is, how will you eat yours?"

Recipe contributed by: Dr Britt Cordi, www.brittsuperfoods.com

VEGETARIAN EASTER ENERGY EGGS

Looking for a delicious Easter treat that doesn't make you feel guilty? Then try our wheatgrass, ginger and turmeric energy easter eggs!

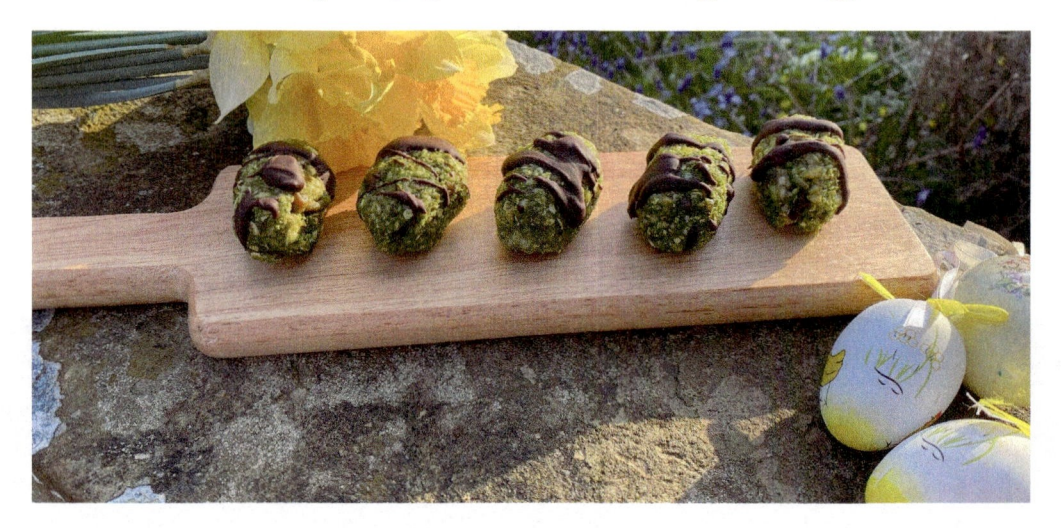

Ingredients

- 200g dates(pitted)
- 200g cashews(toasted)
- 50g oats
- 1 tbsp. coconut oil
- 1 sachet Britt's superfoods wheatgrass juice
- 1 sachet Britt's superfoods ginger, turmeric and apple juice
- dark chocolate for drizzle

Directions

1. Start by soaking the dates in warm water for 10 mins to soften, then drain. Add all ingredients except chocolate to a processor and mix until combined.

2. Form into egg-shaped pieces and place on baking paper on a tray and put into the fridge until hard.

3. Melt chocolate and drizzle over the top of eggs and place back in the fridge to harden.

4. Check back tomorrow for results and to see the energy eggs that give you a guilt free Easter treat

Recipe contributed by: Dr Britt Cordi, www.brittsuperfoods.com

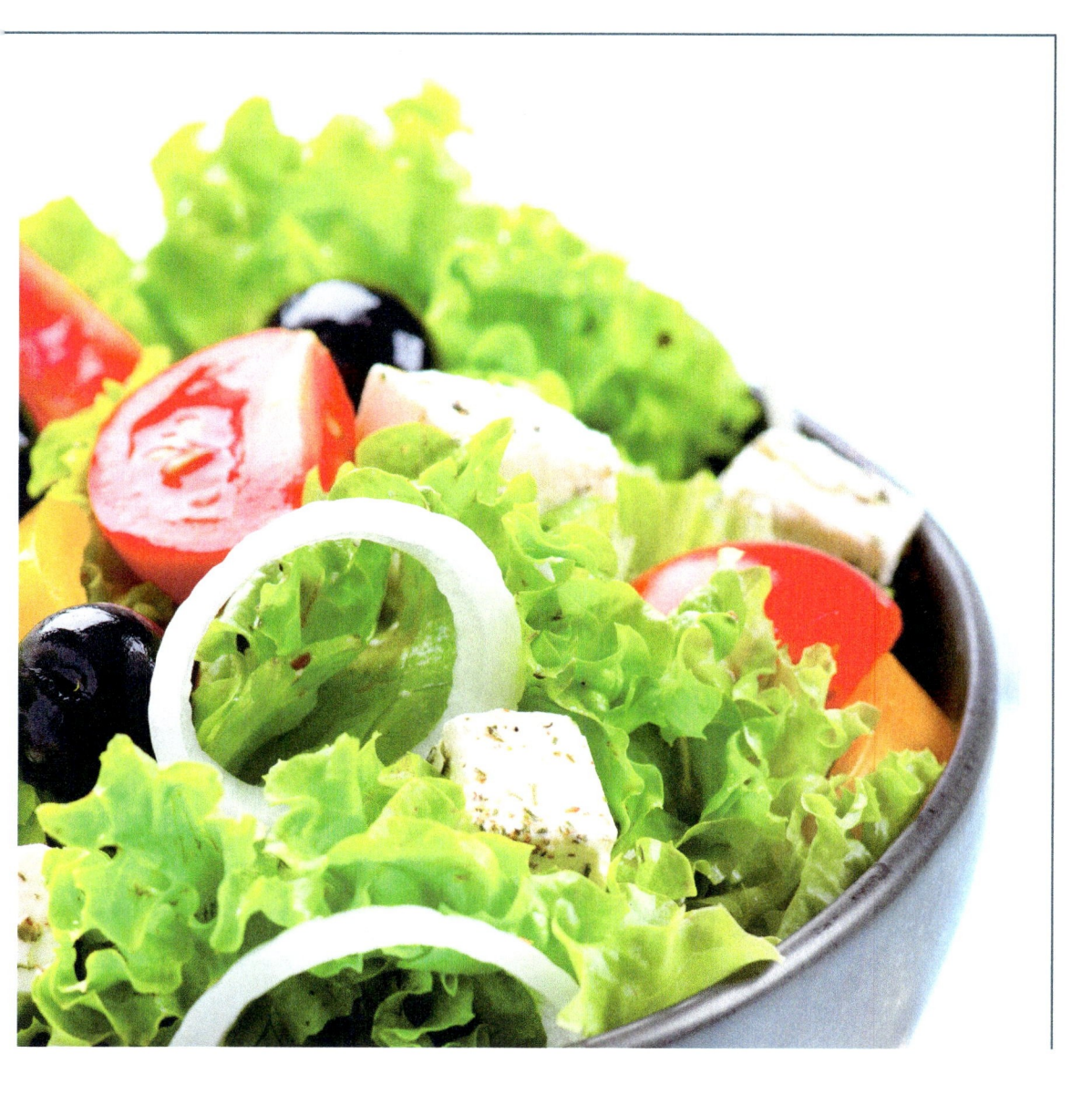

SALADS AND SIDES

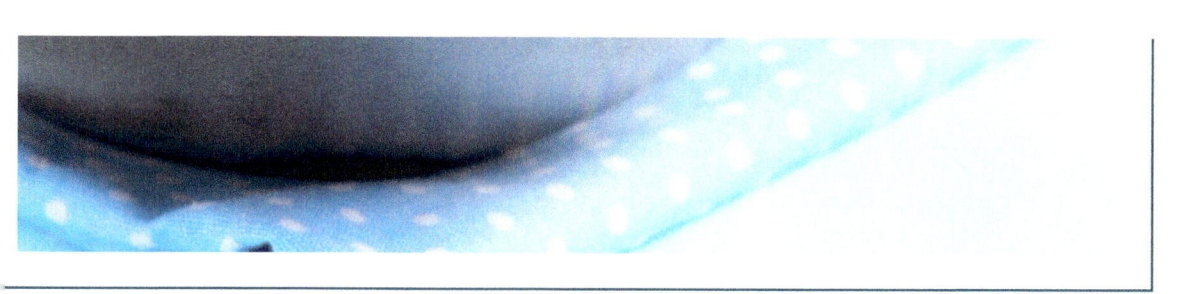

FRESH GREEK SALAD (DAIRY-FREE)

A crunchy mix of raw vegetables, ideal for summer, rich in antioxidants, Vitamin C, Vitamin K and fibre.

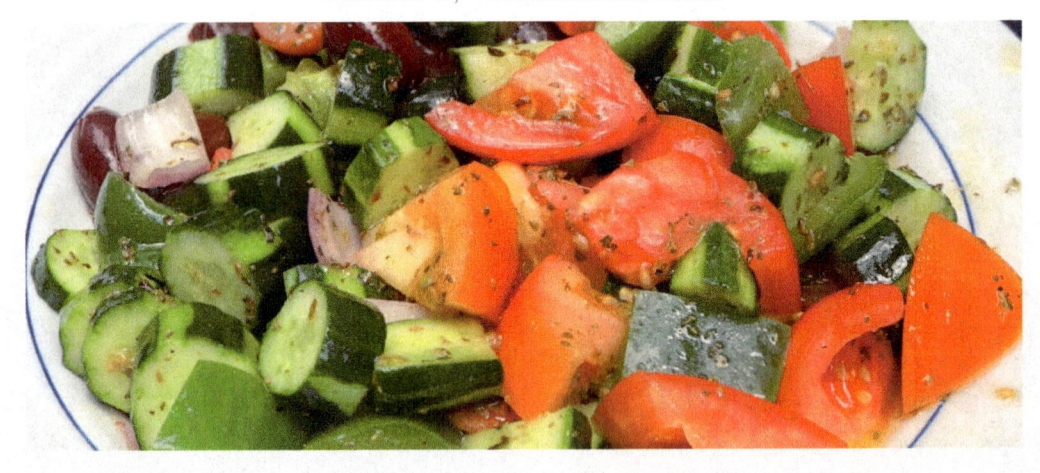

Ingredients

- 1 cucumber
- 1 small purple onion
- 4 halved cherry tomatoes or 1 large diced tomato
- ½ bell pepper diced
- 1 handful of Kalamata olives (pits removed)
- dried oregano
- salt and black pepper
- extra virgin olive oil
- squeeze of lemon

Directions

1. Mix together in a bowl 1 cucumber diced into 1-inch chunks, 1 small purple onion sliced, 4 halved cherry tomatoes or 1 large diced tomato, ½ bell pepper diced, and a handful of Kalamata olives (pits removed).

2. Sprinkle with dried oregano, salt and black pepper to taste.

3. Drizzle with extra virgin olive oil.

4. Finish off with a squeeze of lemon.

Recipe contributed by: The Cancer Coach, www.thecancercoach.org

PEA AND LETTUCE SOUP

Whether it's too cold for lots of salads, or you're after a light summer supper, this delicious and vibrant green soup is a great way to use up the lettuce in the back of your fridge.

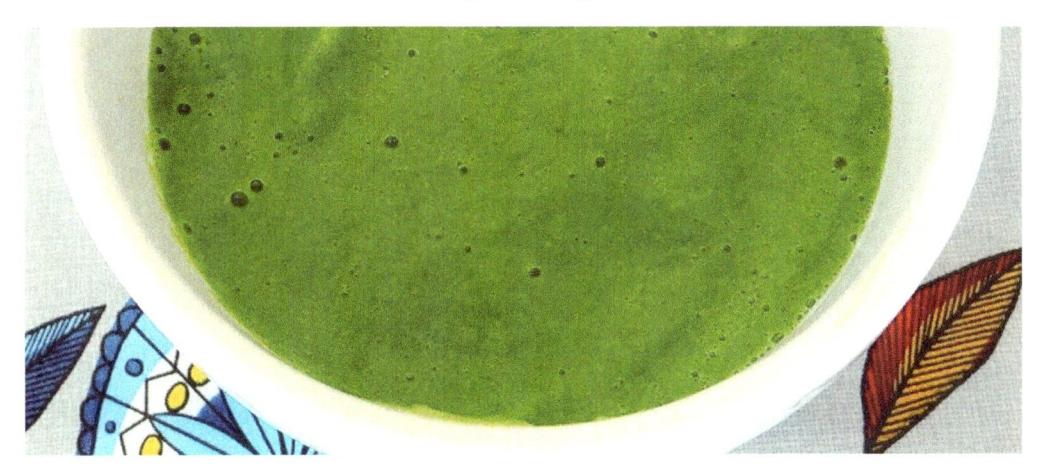

Ingredients

- 1 leek
- 1 head of lettuce
- 2 handfuls garden peas – add, plus any extra water needed
- 2 scoops of pea or faba bean protein powder (optional)
- 1 extra low salt organic stock cube
- Freshly grated nutmeg and seasoning to taste

Directions

1. Finely chop the leek and simmer in a little coconut oil till soft.

2. Chop and add the lettuce.

3. Add the peas, plus enough water to cover.

4. Stir in the pea protein powder (optional), nutmeg, seasoning and stock cube.

5. When hot, blend and serve – with optional garnish (lemon zest is nice on this one).

And there are usually some peas somewhere in the back of the freezer, so you may not have to think about getting extra ingredients in. It's not only super-quick and convenient, it's also rich in vitamin C, plant fibre and a range of nutrients that are great for your liver and immune system.

Recipe contributed by: Kirsten Chick (kirstenchick.com)

PRAWN AND BLUEBERRY SALAD WITH TANGY AVOCADO SAUCE

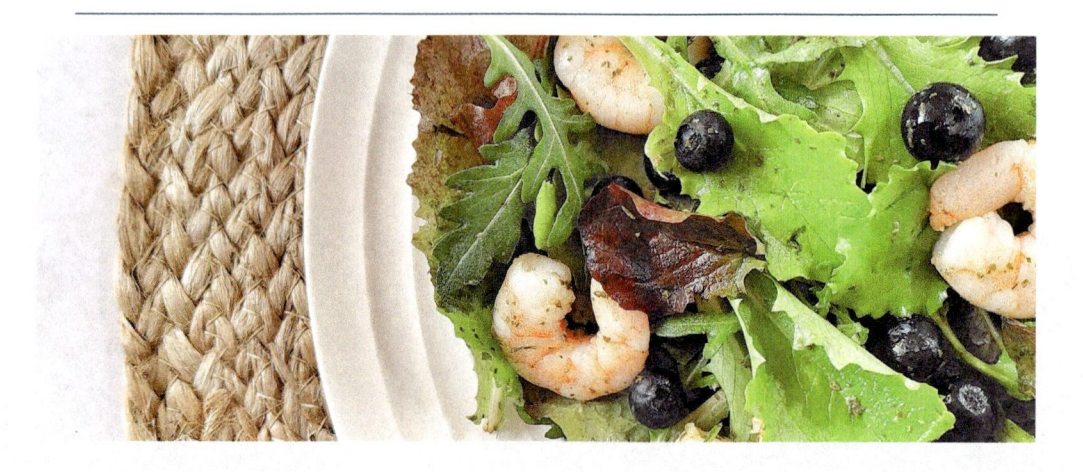

Ingredients

Salad

- 150g cooked prawns
- 55g baby leaf and rocket salad
- 125g blueberries
- 1 tbsp. Tangy Avocado Sauce

Tangy Avocado Sauce

- 2 ripe avocados, halved and pitted
- Juice of 1 lime (2 tablespoons)
- 1 tbsp. apple cider vinegar
- 3 garlic cloves, smashed
- ½ tsp. sea salt
- 60g fresh flat-leaf parsley with stems
- 120ml olive oil, plus more if needed

Directions

1. First, make the dressing: Scoop out the avocado flesh into a food processor. Add the lime juice, vinegar, salt and parsley and process to combine.

2. With the motor running, slowly add the olive oil through the feed tube (adding more as required) until the desired consistency is reached.

3. Next, make the salad. Place the salad ingredients and the dressing in a large bowl.

4. Toss gently and serve.

Top tips:
- *Be sure to use a mild-tasting olive oil so as not to overpower the flavour of the other ingredients.*
- *Substituting 20g of dried parsley for 60g of fresh works well, too.*

Recipe contributed by: Chi Feasey, https://chifeasey.com/

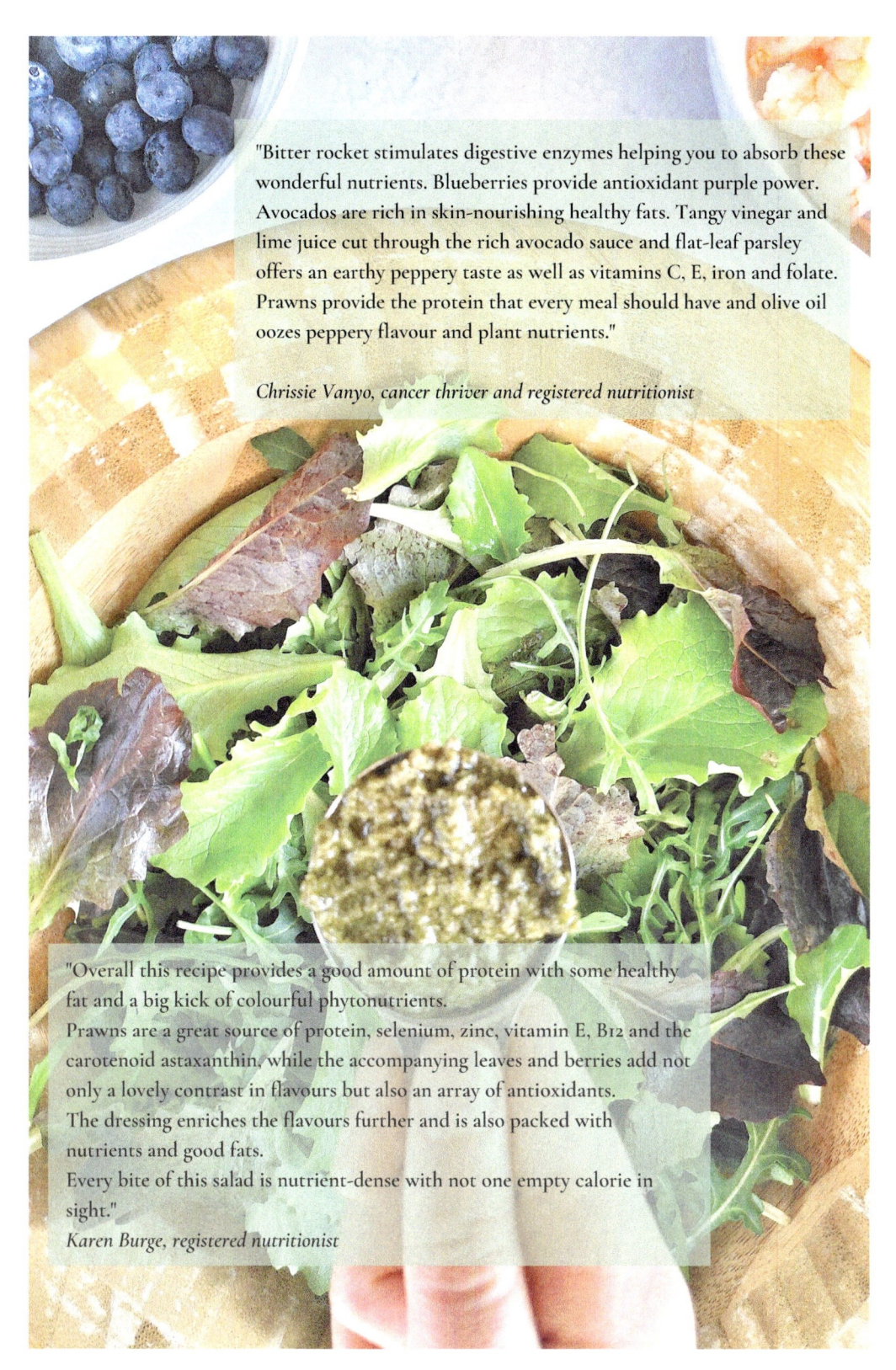

"Bitter rocket stimulates digestive enzymes helping you to absorb these wonderful nutrients. Blueberries provide antioxidant purple power. Avocados are rich in skin-nourishing healthy fats. Tangy vinegar and lime juice cut through the rich avocado sauce and flat-leaf parsley offers an earthy peppery taste as well as vitamins C, E, iron and folate. Prawns provide the protein that every meal should have and olive oil oozes peppery flavour and plant nutrients."

Chrissie Vanyo, cancer thriver and registered nutritionist

"Overall this recipe provides a good amount of protein with some healthy fat and a big kick of colourful phytonutrients.
Prawns are a great source of protein, selenium, zinc, vitamin E, B12 and the carotenoid astaxanthin, while the accompanying leaves and berries add not only a lovely contrast in flavours but also an array of antioxidants.
The dressing enriches the flavours further and is also packed with nutrients and good fats.
Every bite of this salad is nutrient-dense with not one empty calorie in sight."
Karen Burge, registered nutritionist

PRAWN AND MANGO SALAD

A fresh mango flavour salad for any occasion.

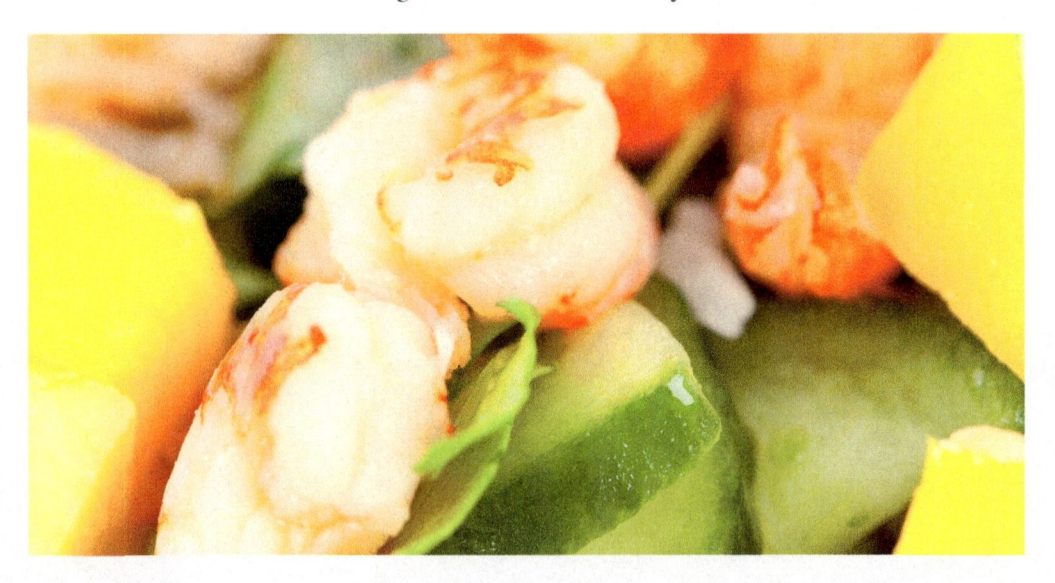

Ingredients

- 200g white or savoy cabbage
- 1 large carrot
- 1 avocado
- 250g king prawns (defrosted if frozen)
- Slice of mango
- White wine vinegar
- Olive oil,
- Salt and pepper

Directions

1. Finely chop the cabbage and carrot.
2. Quarter, pit and peel the avocado; cube.
3. Dice the mango, and add to the veg with the prawns.
4. Dress with oil and vinegar; season.

NB: Also good with diced chicken and balsamic vinegar.

Recipe contributed by: Jenny Phillips, www.inspirednutrition.co.uk

A SIDE OF VITAMIN C

Did you know that red bell peppers have about three times as much vitamin C as oranges? This lovely side dish works well with roasted chicken or poached fish.

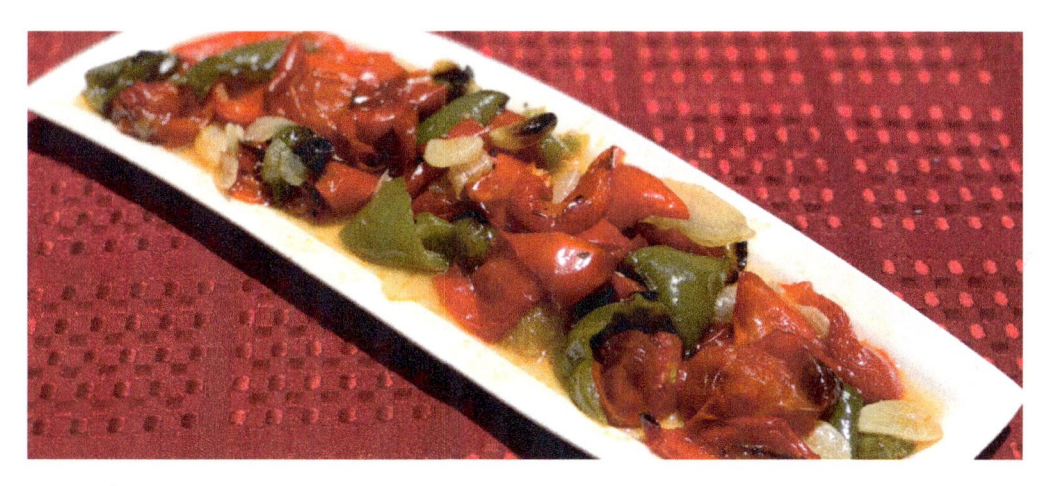

Ingredients

- 1 green and 3 red bell peppers, cut into cubes, seeds and stems removed
- 10-12 whole cherry tomatoes
- 1 large white onion cut into chunks
- 1 head of garlic — cloves separated, peeled, and cut in half

Directions

1. Preheat oven to 180C.
2. Toss together all ingredients in a bowl.
3. Drizzle with 1 tablespoon olive oil, season with salt and pepper and toss gently.
4. Place everything onto a large baking sheet with sides
5. Bake in oven 25 to 30 minutes until onions are golden, tomatoes begin to burst, and peppers are soft.
6. Serve warm or at room temperature.

Recipe contributed by: The Cancer Coach, www.thecancercoach.org

ALL GREEN QUINOA SALAD

It's no secret that quinoa is considered a superfood for its array of antioxidants, vitamins and minerals. This gluten-free seed is a delicious protein source and is low in carbs.

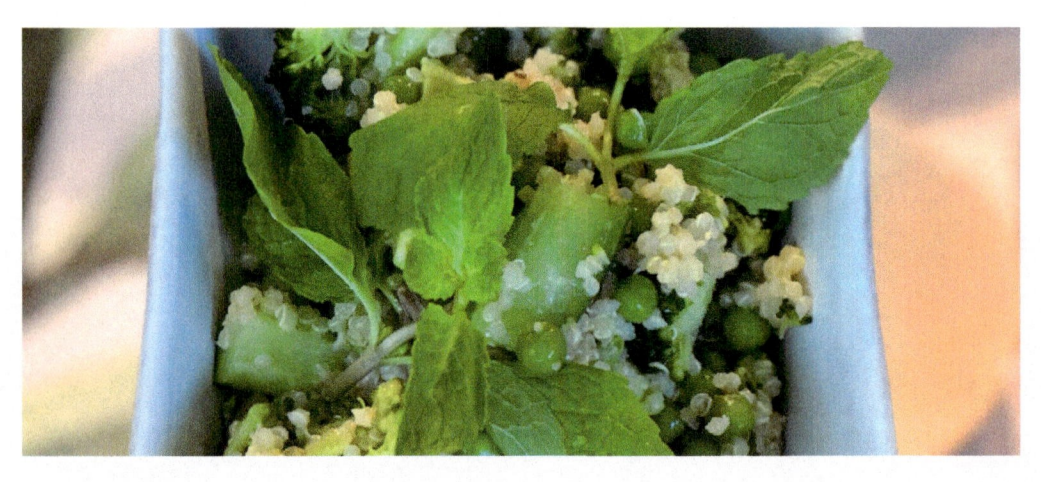

Ingredients

- 2 cups cooked quinoa
- 1 avocado, diced
- ½ cup green peas, cooked (you can use salt-free, frozen peas)
- 1 crown broccoli, cut into florets, slightly steamed, but still crunchy
- 1 cucumber, diced
- 2 tablespoons mint, chopped
- 2 tablespoons sunflower seeds

Directions

1. Toss quinoa, avocado, peas, broccoli, cucumber, and mint into a large bowl.
2. Mix gently.
3. Top with sunflower seeds and serve.
4. Add squeeze of lemon or lime juice if you desire just before serving.

Recipe contributed by: The Cancer Coach, www.thecancercoach.org

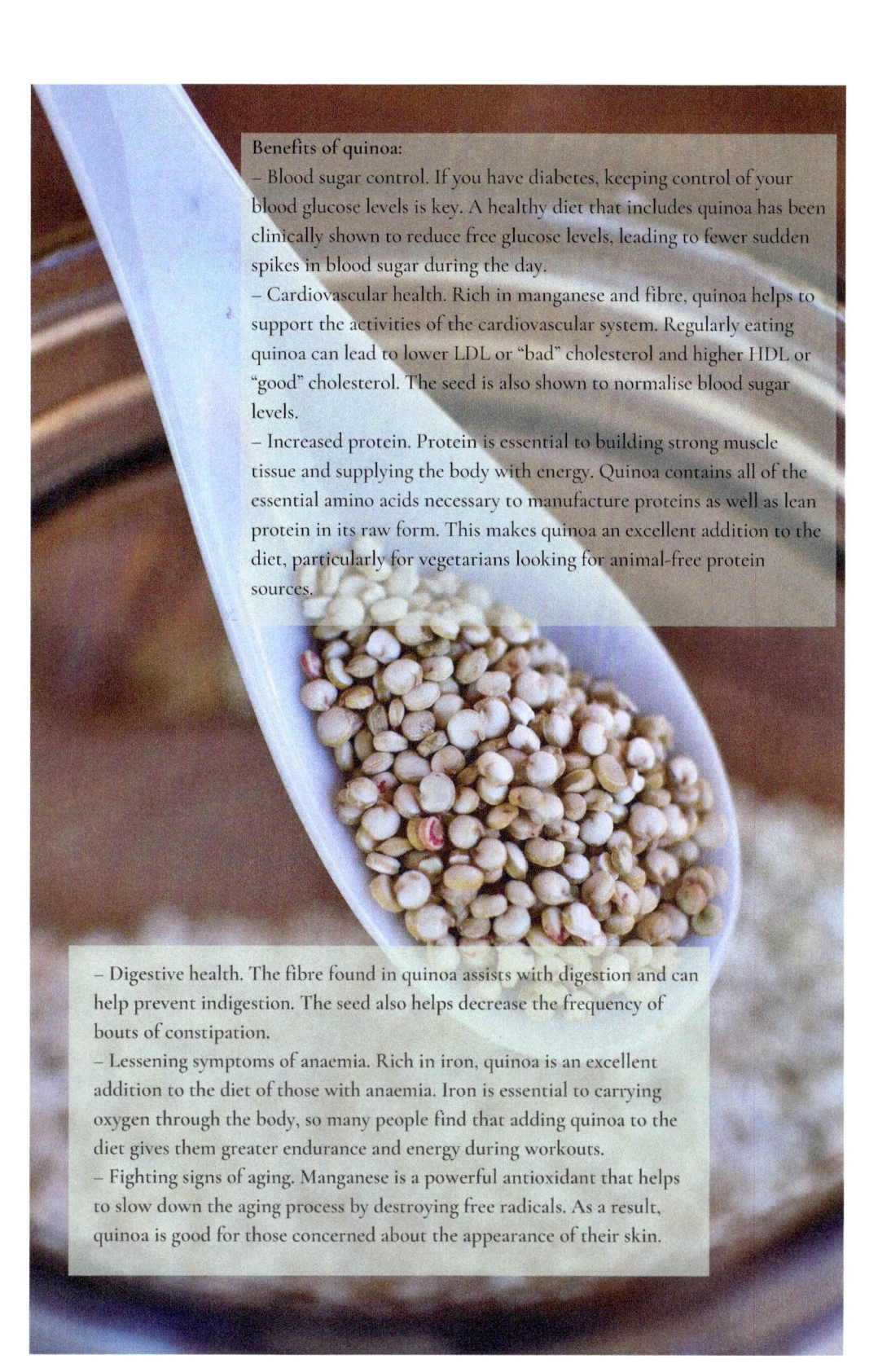

Benefits of quinoa:
– Blood sugar control. If you have diabetes, keeping control of your blood glucose levels is key. A healthy diet that includes quinoa has been clinically shown to reduce free glucose levels, leading to fewer sudden spikes in blood sugar during the day.
– Cardiovascular health. Rich in manganese and fibre, quinoa helps to support the activities of the cardiovascular system. Regularly eating quinoa can lead to lower LDL or "bad" cholesterol and higher HDL or "good" cholesterol. The seed is also shown to normalise blood sugar levels.
– Increased protein. Protein is essential to building strong muscle tissue and supplying the body with energy. Quinoa contains all of the essential amino acids necessary to manufacture proteins as well as lean protein in its raw form. This makes quinoa an excellent addition to the diet, particularly for vegetarians looking for animal-free protein sources.

– Digestive health. The fibre found in quinoa assists with digestion and can help prevent indigestion. The seed also helps decrease the frequency of bouts of constipation.
– Lessening symptoms of anaemia. Rich in iron, quinoa is an excellent addition to the diet of those with anaemia. Iron is essential to carrying oxygen through the body, so many people find that adding quinoa to the diet gives them greater endurance and energy during workouts.
– Fighting signs of aging. Manganese is a powerful antioxidant that helps to slow down the aging process by destroying free radicals. As a result, quinoa is good for those concerned about the appearance of their skin.

SIMPLE STOVETOP VEGGIES

Tired of the same-old week night veggies? This quick side dish mixes it up a bit and works for any meal. Remember the more colorful the selection of veggies, the better.

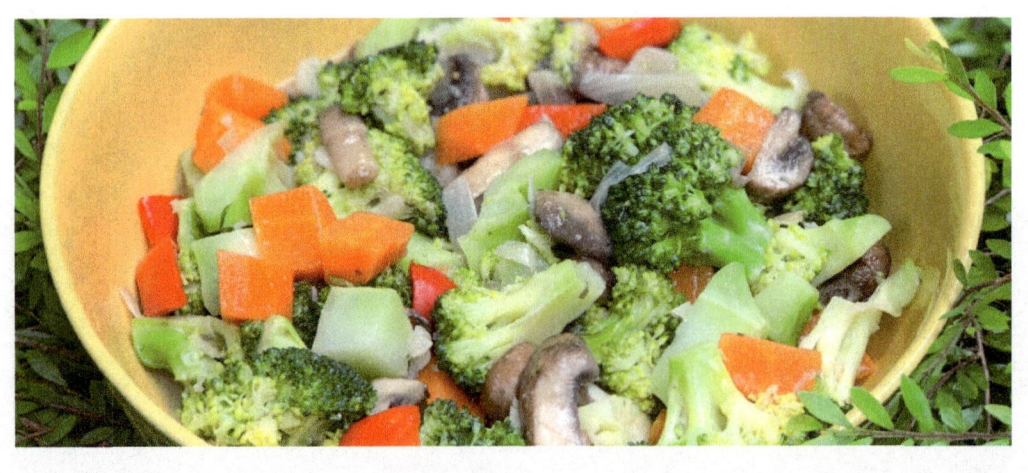

Ingredients

- 3 tsp. extra virgin olive oil
- 1 bulb garlic, thinly sliced
- 1 onion, diced small
- 1 broccoli crown, cut into small florets
- 1 carrot, diced small
- 1 red bell pepper, diced small
- 4 mushrooms, thinly sliced
- 1/2 cup of chicken bone broth*
- 2 teaspoons salt
- black pepper (freshly ground)

Directions

1. Heat oil in a wok or large skillet with deep sides.

2. Add onion and garlic and cook for 1-2 minutes until fragrant and starting to soften.

3. Add vegetables and mix with aromatics. Carefully add ½ cup of water; it will splatter and steam.

4. As water cooks off and veggies begin to soften add 1 cup of chicken broth and stir.

5. Cook until vegetables are soft, but not mushy.

*Buy chicken broth made from real chicken bones (choose organic). Avoid using chicken stock cubes containing artificial chemicals.

Recipe contributed by: The Cancer Coach, www.thecancercoach.org

ROASTED CAULIFLOWER INDIAN STYLE

The humble cauliflower lights up with a beautiful mix of Indian spices.

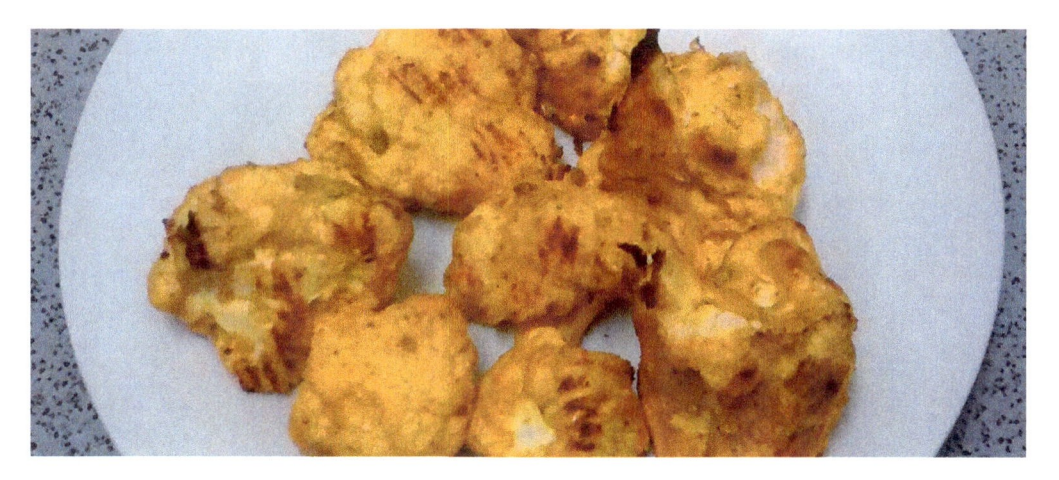

Ingredients

- One cauliflower head
- 250 gr Greek yogurt, full fat
- 2 garlic cloves, minced
- 1 tsp. turmeric powder
- 1 tsp. cumin powder
- Few fresh coriander leaves, finely chopped
- Few fresh curry leaves, finely chopped
- ¼ tsp. cinnamon powder
- ¼ tsp. clove powder
- ½ (tsp.??) curry madras powder
- ½ tsp. red chili flakes
- ½ tsp. paprika or Cayenne pepper
- Juice of half lemon or one lime
- Pinch of good quality sea salt

Directions

1. Preheat the oven 190°
2. Lay an oven tray with baking paper.
3. Gently break the cauliflower into florets, wash them thoroughly and set aside.
4. In a bowl, mix all the herbs and spices.
5. Add the lemon juice and the yogurt and mix well.
6. Take one cauliflower floret, dip it in the spicy yogurt, coat it well, place it on the baking tray.
7. Repeat with all the florets.
8. Place the tray in the oven and bake for 25-30 minutes, until the florets are golden.

Enjoy!

Recipe contributed by: Silvia Mensurati, www.nutritiontoheal.com

ROASTED BUTTERNUT AND POMEGRANATE SALAD

Packed with nutrients and full of flavour, this dish is sure to impress your guests; the sweetness of the caramelized butternut and onion marries perfectly with the tangy crunchiness of the pomegranate and green leaves.

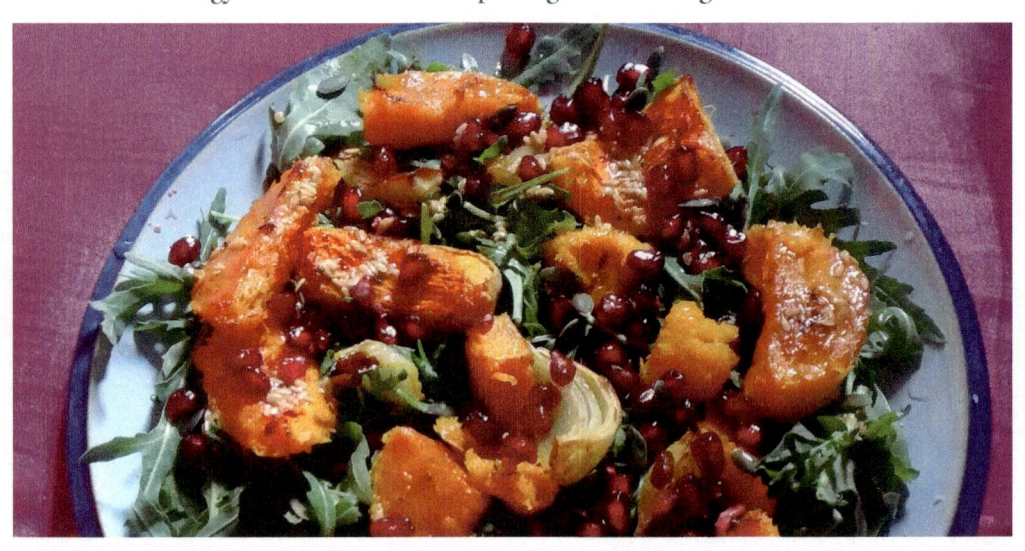

Ingredients

- One butternut squash, washed, deseeded and cut into 1/2 inch slices
- 1 onion, peeled and cut in chunks
- 1 tbsp. good quality extra virgin olive oil
- ½ tsp. paprika
- ½ tsp. red chilli
- A couple of drops of organic Canadian maple syrup or good quality organic honey
- Rocket salad
- Seeds of one pomegranate
- 1 tbsp. pumpkin seeds
- 1 tbsp. linseeds or/and sesame seeds

For the dressing

- 2 tbsp. good quality extra virgin olive oil
- Juice of a small lime
- ½ tbsp. ground flax seeds
- ½ tsp. good quality sea salt
- ¼ tsp. freshly ground black pepper

Recipe contributed by: Silvia Mensurati, www.nutritiontoheal.com

Directions

1. Preheat oven to 180 degrees

2. In an oven dish, gently toss the butternut squash and onion with the extra virgin olive oil, maple syrup, chilli and paprika.

3. Roast for 35-40 minutes until the squash has softened with golden edges. Set aside.

4. Mix together all the dressing ingredients and set aside.

5. Wash the rocket leaves and arrange them on a serving plate.

6. Place the roasted butternut on top, add the pomegranate, pumpkin and linseeds, pour the dressing over and voilà, ready!

Serve warm and enjoy

Leave the peel of the squash on during roasting for added flavour, plus it is so much easier to remove when cooked. Make sure to buy organic!

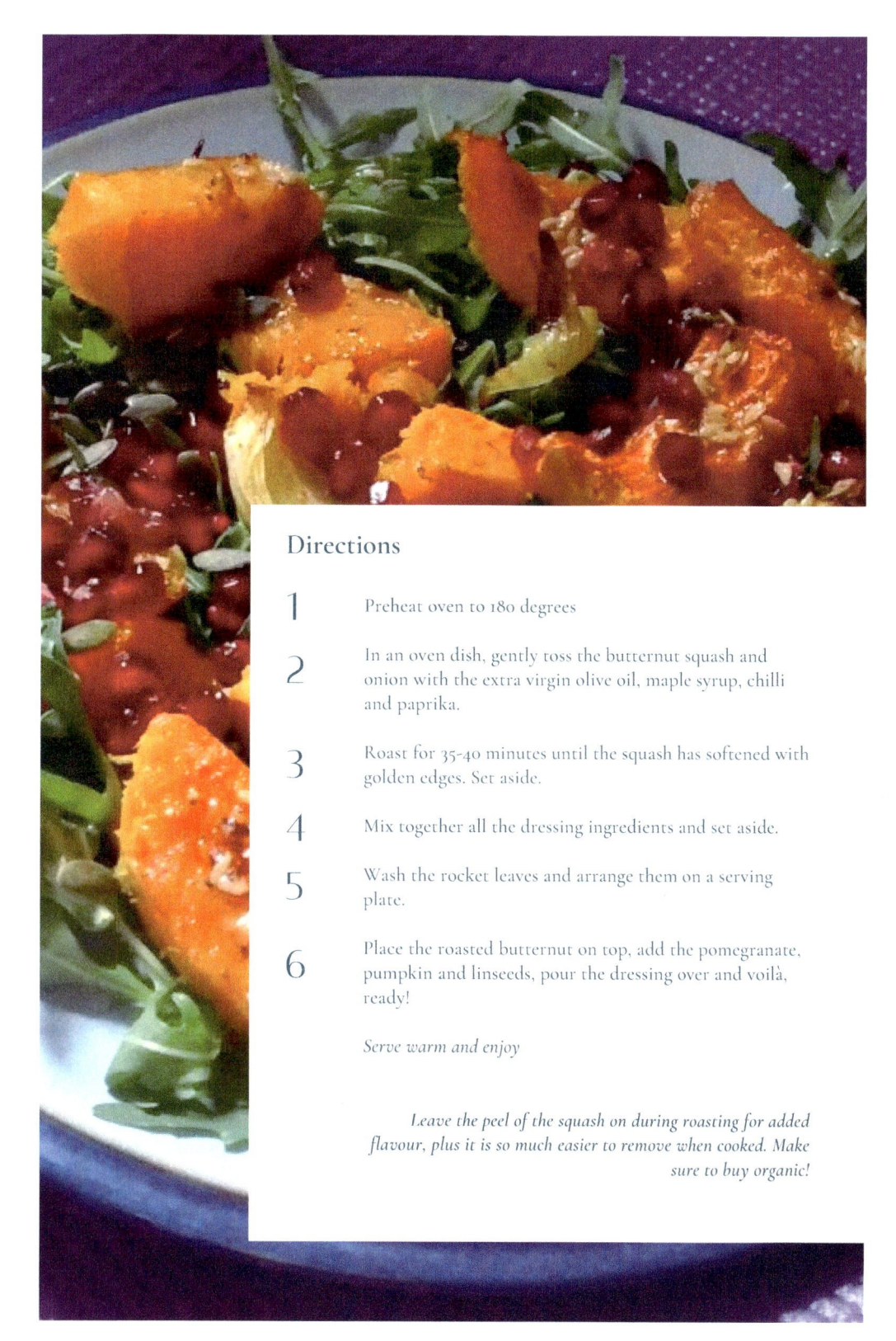

MISO ROASTED MUSHROOMS AND SPRING ONIONS WITH JAPANESE TAMARI SUPERSEEDS

This delicious recipe works beautifully as a hearty side dish. Or, double the amount and make it your main.

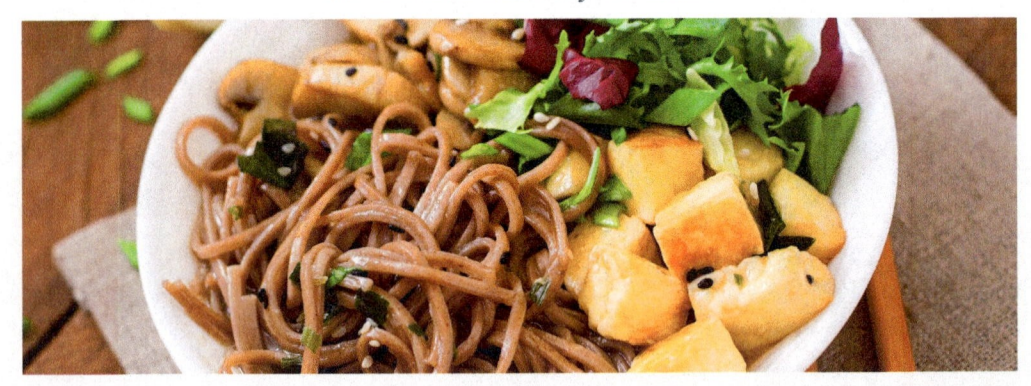

Ingredients

- 1 pack/box brown cup mushrooms
- 1 bunch of spring onions
- 1 heaped tbsp. brown rice miso paste
- 1 tsp. cider vinegar
- 1 tbsp. coconut oil (melted)
- 1 tsp. sesame oil
- Juice of ¼ lemon
- 2x tbsp. Japanese Tamari Superseeds

Directions

1. Set the oven to 200°C.

2. Chop the mushrooms into halves and the spring onions into inch-long chunks, keeping the leafy bits for later.

3. Mix all the dressing ingredients in a bowl. Add the mushrooms and spring onions and mix using your hands before transferring to a baking tray.

4. Roast for 20 - 30 mins. To get them nice and crispy you may want to drain some of the liquid 15 mins in and switch to a grill setting for the last 5 mins.

5. Remove and transfer to a plate.

6. Finish with a sprinkle of the finely chopped spring onion leaves and Japanese Tamari Superseeds.

Recipe from Food for Life series, Yes to Life

JERK CHICKEN SALAD

Salad with style

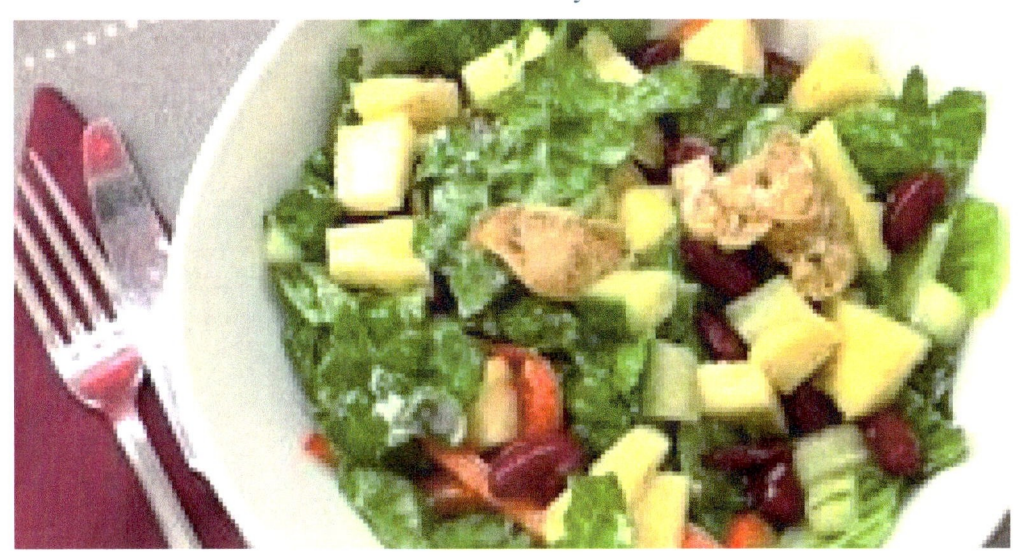

Ingredients

- 1 tbsp. olive oil
- 1 tbsp. jerk seasoning
- 450g skinless chicken thighs, cut into strips
- 1 large romaine lettuce
- ½ medium pineapple, diced
- 1 red pepper thinly sliced
- 3 inch cucumber, diced
- 1 can red kidney beans
- 1 lime
- 100ml plain yoghurt
- 2 tsp. maple syrup

Directions

1. In a bowl, mix the jerk seasoning and olive oil. Add the chicken and mix well to coat the chicken.

2. Bake the chicken for 30 minutes at 200°C, or until cooked.

3. Wash and shred the lettuce, line a salad bowl.

4. Mix through the pineapple, red pepper and cucumber. Add the kidney beans and mix well.

5. To make the dressing, zest the lime and add 1 tsp. to the yoghurt along with the juice of half the fruit. Mix well and stir in maple syrup to taste.

6. Add the hot chicken to the salad, top with dressing and mix well.

Recipe contributed by: Jenny Phillips, www.inspirednutrition.co.uk

KALE AND SWEET POTATO CHIPS

A quick and easy recipe for some super-healthy and crispy chips.

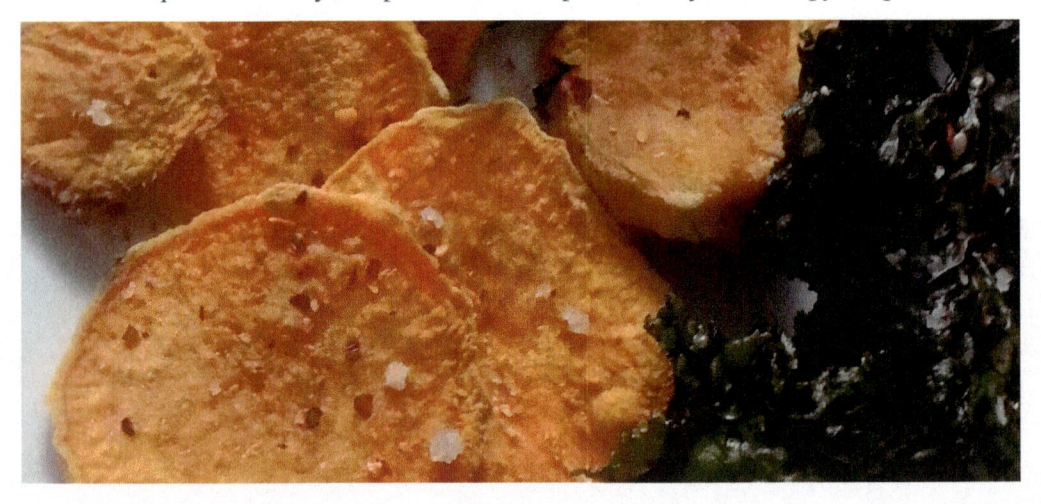

Ingredients

- 1 medium sweet potato or 2 small ones
- 4 large kale leaves
- 2 tbsp. organic extra virgin olive oil
- ½ tsp. red chilli flakes
- ½ tsp. sesame seeds
- Good quality sea salt, for seasoning

Directions

1. Preheat the oven to 190°C, 170° fan, 375°F.
2. Peel the sweet potato, slice it into thins and put it in a small bowl.
3. Drizzle with a tbsp. of extra virgin olive oil and mix well.
4. Arrange the sweet potato thins in a single layer on a parchment-lined baking sheet, making sure they don't overlap.
5. Bake the sweet potato thins for 10 minutes (temp??), turn them over, and keep baking for 8-10 minutes more, until crisp. Season with good quality sea salt.
6. Wash the kale thoroughly, gently break the leaves into small pieces and put these in a small bowl.
7. Drizzle with a tbsp. of extra virgin olive oil, add a pinch of red chilli flakes and massage the leaves so that they are well coated.

Recipe contributed by: Silvia Mensurati, www.nutritiontoheal.com

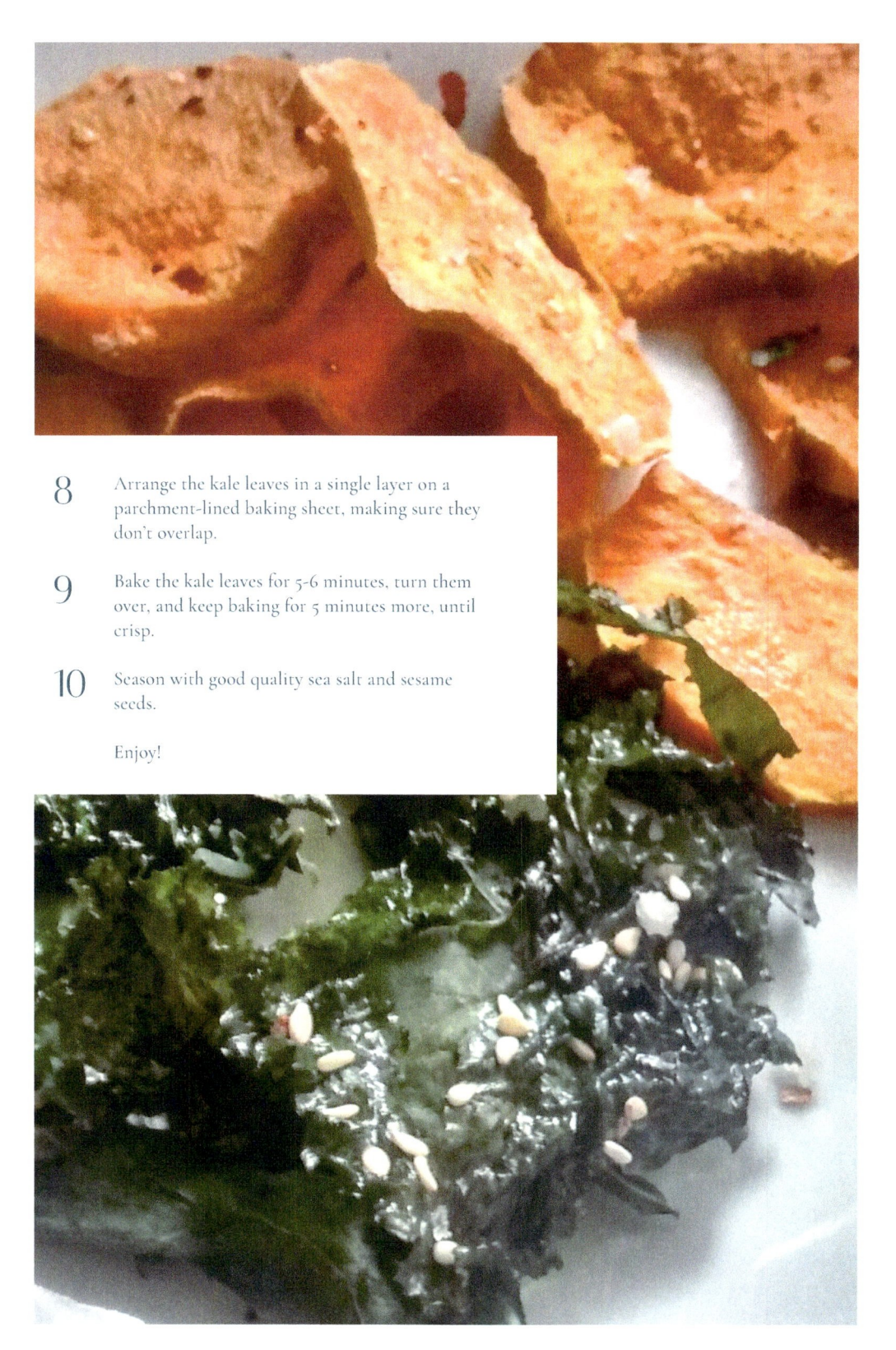

8. Arrange the kale leaves in a single layer on a parchment-lined baking sheet, making sure they don't overlap.

9. Bake the kale leaves for 5-6 minutes, turn them over, and keep baking for 5 minutes more, until crisp.

10. Season with good quality sea salt and sesame seeds.

Enjoy!

TUNA MIX WRAPS

Enjoy this delicious dish for breakfast or lunch!

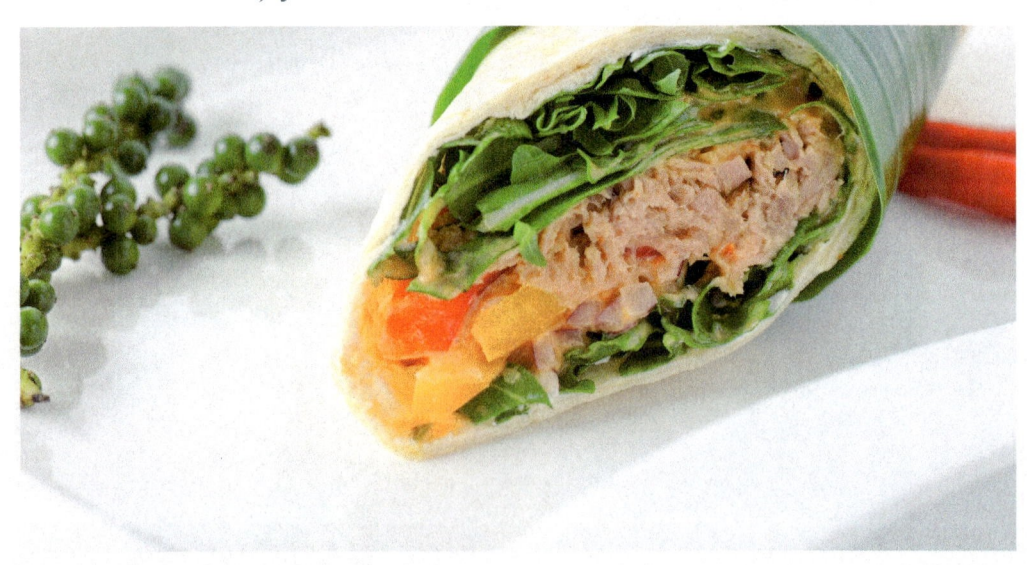

Ingredients

- 1 bunch organic romaine lettuce (or spinach, stalks removed)
- 1 avocado, sliced
- 3 spring onions, chopped
- 1 red/orange bell pepper, chopped
- 1-cup sweet corn
- ½ lime
- 1 tbsp. extra virgin olive oil
- Pinch of salt and black pepper
- 20 gms tuna, steamed or baked (canned tuna in spring water is fine)
- Handful coriander, chopped

Directions

1. Wash the lettuce, dry and remove stem from the middle.
2. Put all vegetables in a bowl.
3. With a fork, break the tuna into small pieces and add to veggies.
4. Add the lime juice, olive oil and coriander, mix together thoroughly.
5. Place one or two lettuce leaves on a plate, scoop a good amount of tuna mix onto the leaves.
6. Top with avocado and gently roll the leaves into wraps.

Recipe from Food for Life series, Yes to Life

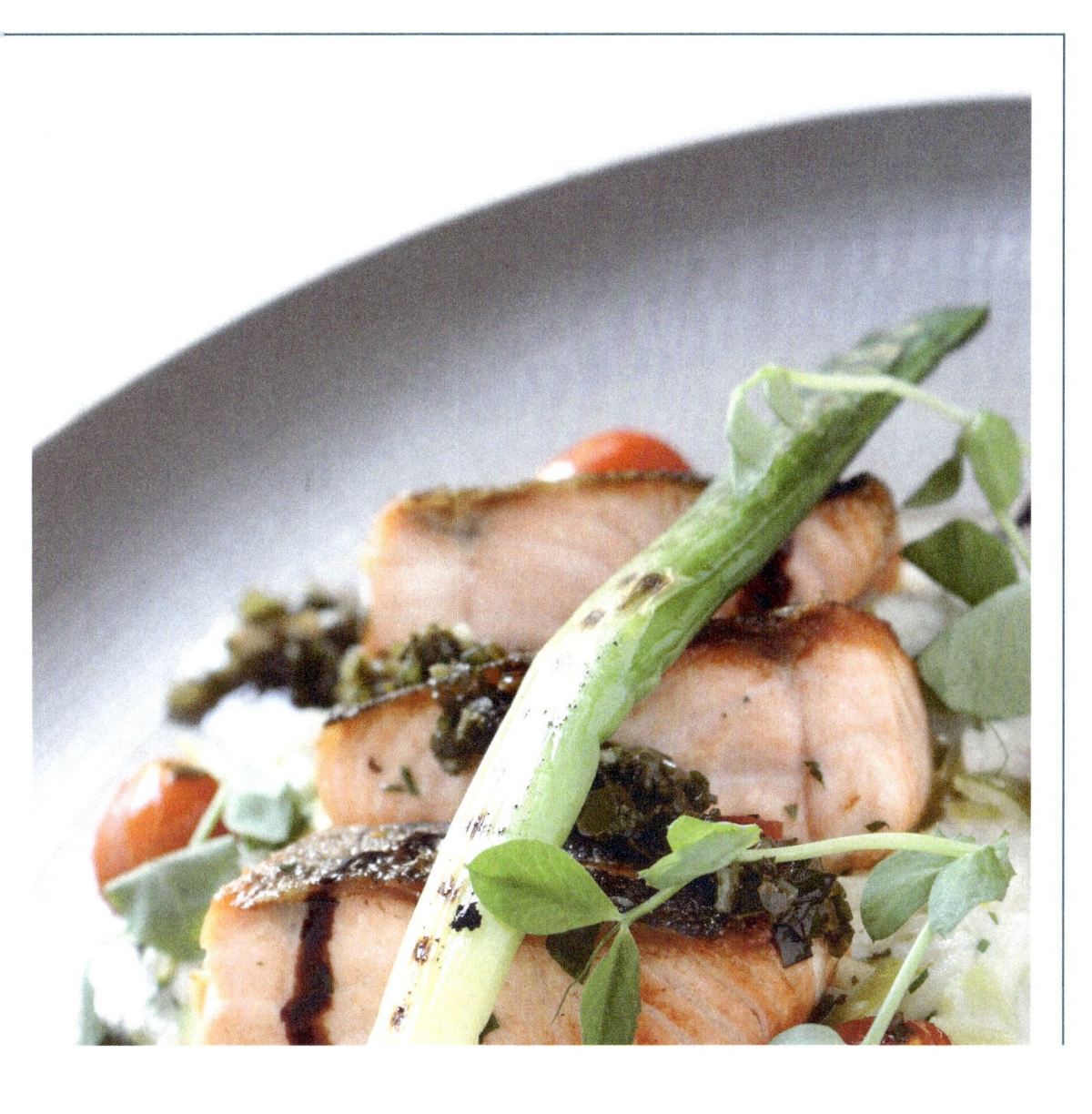

MAINS

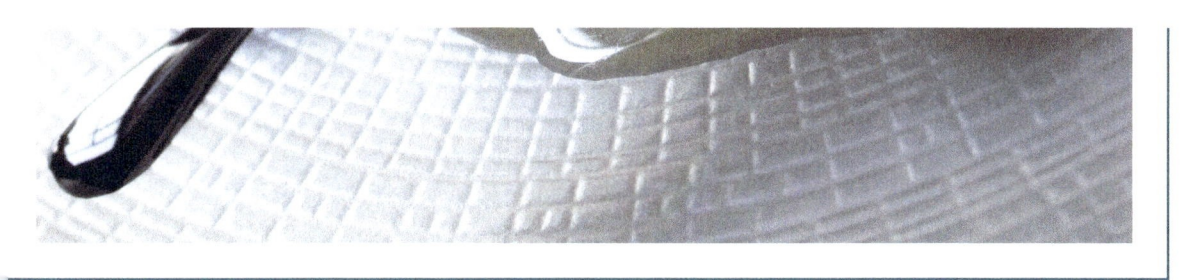

MUSHROOM SOUP

For mushrooms soup lovers.

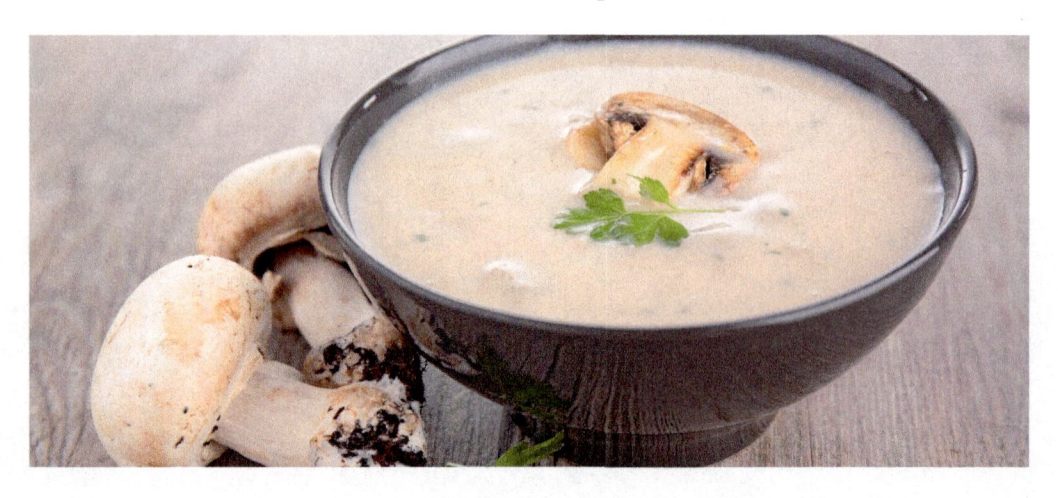

Ingredients

- 500g mushrooms
- 1 large onion, peeled and diced
- 500ml homemade vegetable stock or broth
- 100ml coconut milk
- 1 tbsp. olive oil
- 2 cloves garlic, crushed
- 3-4 sprigs of fresh thyme

Directions

1. Sauté the onions and garlic in the olive oil until soft then add the mushrooms and thyme.

2. Fry the mushrooms until lightly browned, add the hot stock, then pour the contents of the pan into a blender and blend until smooth.

3. Return the soup to the pan, add the coconut milk and heat through.

4. Season to taste and serve in large bowls decorated with a sprig of thyme in each.

Recipe contributed by: Jenny Phillips, www.inspirednutrition.co.uk

VEGAN KALE PESTO

Nutrient rich, easy to make and tastes good with everything!

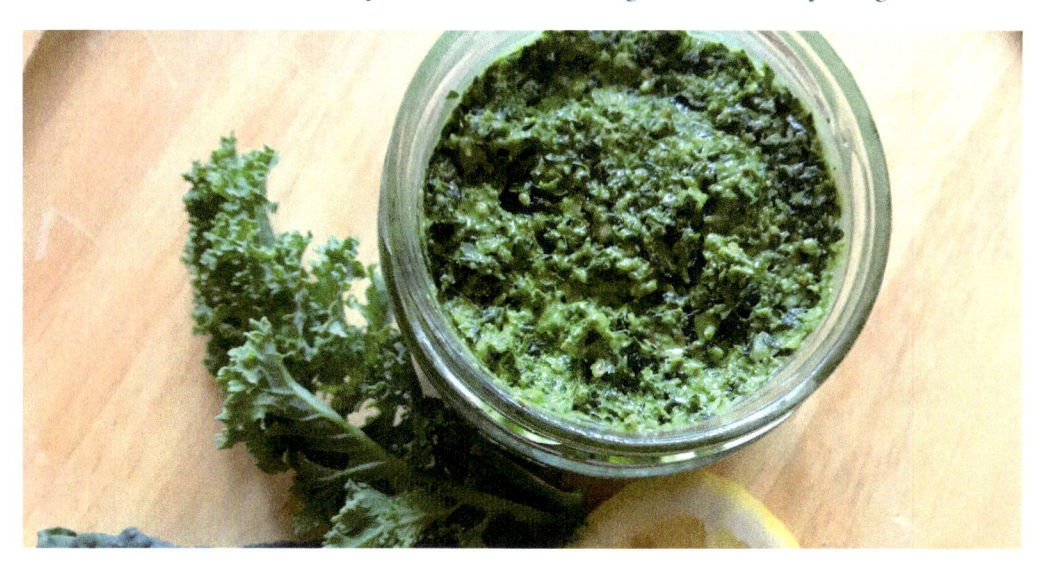

Ingredients

- 2 Britt's Superfoods wheatgrass juice sachets
- Handful of basil
- 3 large garlic cloves
- 2 big handfuls of kale
- 3 tbsp. nuts (we used almonds)
- 1/2 lemon juiced
- 3 tbsp. olive oil
- Salt & pepper to taste

Directions

1. Add everything except the oil into a blender and blitz until fine.
2. Add olive oil to achieve the right consistency.
3. If needed water can be added to make smoother.

Recipe contributed by: Dr Britt Cordi, www.brittsuperfoods.com

ASIAN BAKED FISH PACKETS

A quick, flavorful cooking method that works for almost any fish. The recipe uses individual packets, so you can scale it for a single serving or an entire family. I love to serve this dish when hosting a dinner.

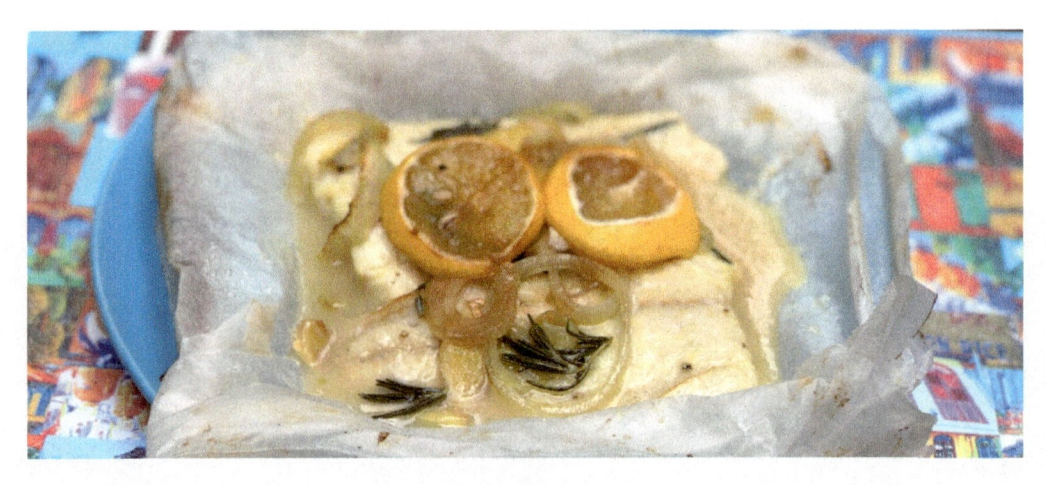

Ingredients

- 1 fish fillet (barramundi, snapper, salmon)
- 3 slices yellow onion
- 2 slices of lemon
- 2 thin slices of ginger
- 1 clove garlic, thinly sliced
- 2 sprigs coriander, leaves and stalks, chopped
- 2 tbsp. water
- 1 tsp. coconut aminos
- 1 tsp. coconut oil
- Salt & pepper

Directions

1. Preheat oven to 200C.
2. Wash fish and pat dry.
3. Take a sheet of baking paper large enough to create a packet for the fish—a little larger than double the fish size.
4. Fold paper in half. Then open it up. Stack in the middle of one half of the paper: onion, lemon, ginger, garlic.
5. Season fish with salt and pepper and place on top of the onion stack. Pour the coconut aminos and coconut oil over the fish. Sprinkle with chopped coriander.
6. Drizzle two tablespoons of water around the outside of the stack. Don't skip the water, this creates steam inside the packet to cook the fish and keep it moist.

Recipe contributed by: The Cancer Coach, www.thecancercoach.org

7 Fold the other half of packet over the top. Working from outside in, turn the edges on top of themselves to form a seal.

8 Make sure this is closed tightly. Continue with additional packets as necessary. Transfer packets to a rimmed baking sheet in a single layer.

9 Do not stack the packets on top of each other.

10 Bake for 10-20 minutes depending on thickness of the fillet.

11 Remove packets from oven and open carefully to allow steam to escape. Serve with a side of steamed vegetables for a complete meal.

Note: You can also use olive oil instead of coconut nut oil + aminos

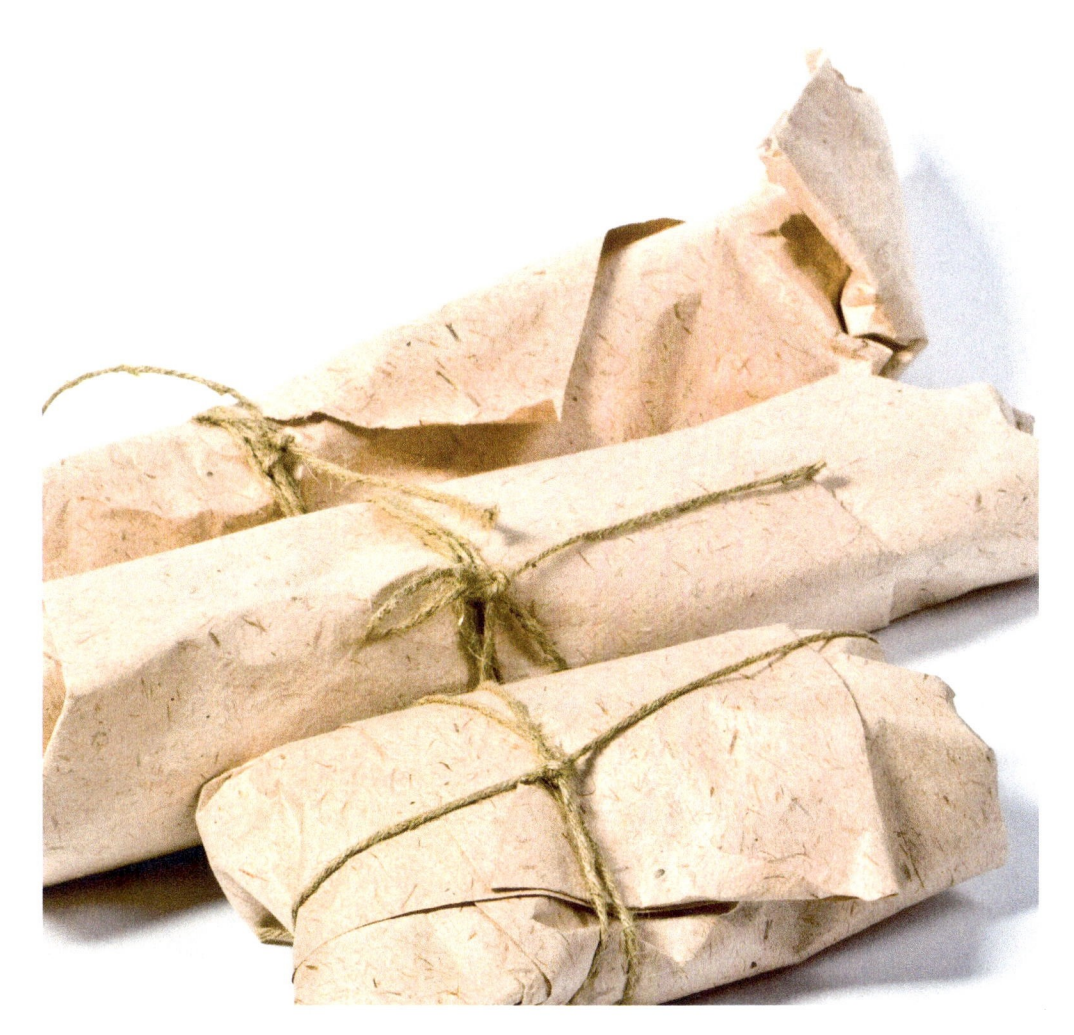

WILD SALMON IN GINGER LEMON MARINADE

Another super-easy, super-quick and super-healthy recipe for you to try! Perfect for busy weeknights, this wild salmon in ginger lemon marinade will be a hit!

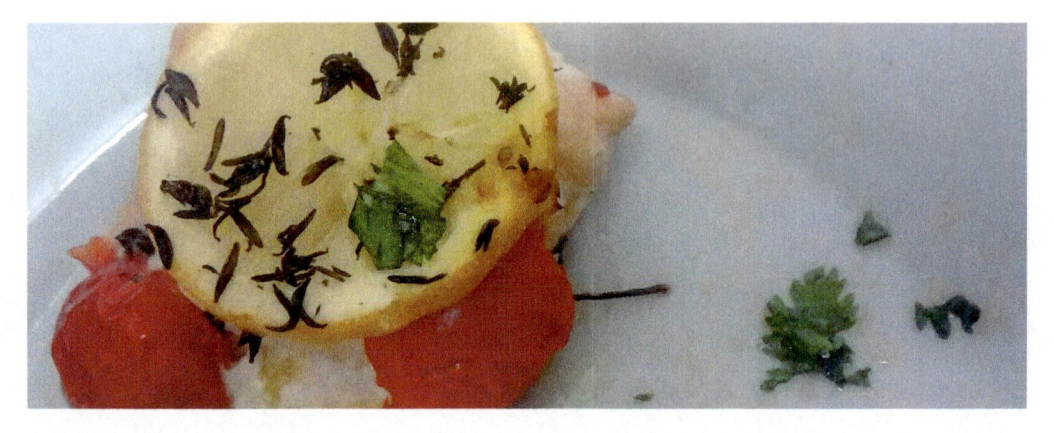

Ingredients

- 4 wild caught salmon fillets
- 1 lemon, sliced
- Few cherry tomatoes

For the marinade

- 1 lime or ½ lemon, juiced
- 1 tsp. grated fresh ginger root
- 2 to 4 cloves garlic, crushed
- Fresh coriander
- Fresh or dried thyme
- Few drops of good quality extra virgin olive oil
- Good quality salt and pepper to taste

Directions

1. Rinse the salmon fillets under running water and place them skin side up in a glass dish.
2. In a glass jar, combine the ingredients for the marinade, seal with a lid and shake vigorously (use a small bowl if you have no jar, and mix well).
3. Pour the marinade over the fillets, ensuring they are fully coated.
4. Cover the dish and let marinate for 30 minutes to 2 hours in the fridge. If you are in a hurry or very hungry, you can skip the fridge time and go straight to the next step.
5. Preheat oven to 180C/160C fan/gas 4.
6. Drain off marinade. Flip salmon to skin side down and place it on chemical- free baking paper.

Recipe contributed by: Silvia Mensurati, www.nutritiontoheal.com

7 Cut the cherry tomatoes in half and place them with the sliced lemon on top of the fillets.

8 Wrap the salmon with the paper and bake for about 15 – 20 minutes, depending on the size of the fillets, until done.

9 If you have no baking paper, simply place the salmon fillets in a glass baking dish to marinade, drain them, and use the same dish for cooking. Grilling is also good!

Enjoy!

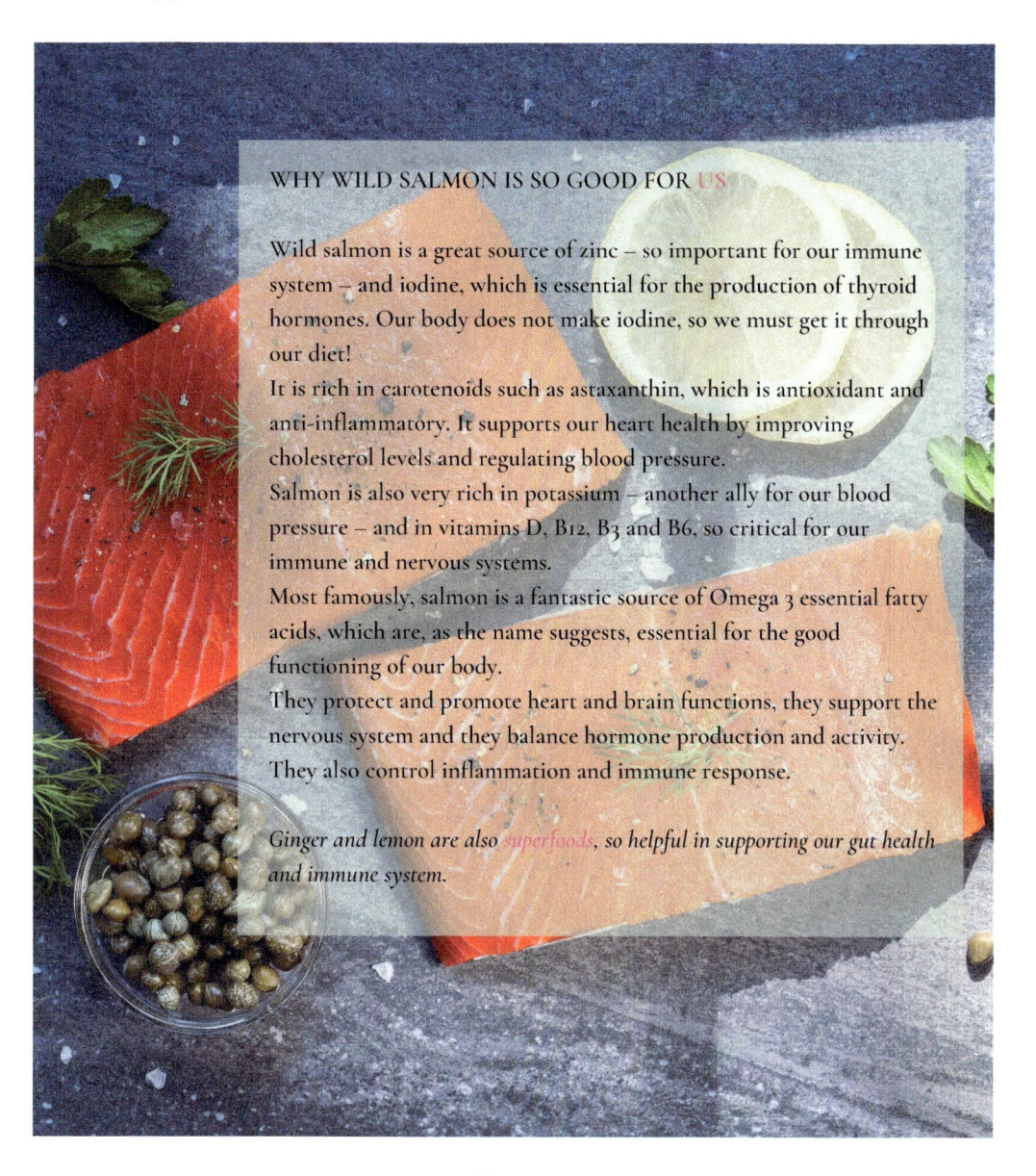

WHY WILD SALMON IS SO GOOD FOR US

Wild salmon is a great source of zinc – so important for our immune system – and iodine, which is essential for the production of thyroid hormones. Our body does not make iodine, so we must get it through our diet!

It is rich in carotenoids such as astaxanthin, which is antioxidant and anti-inflammatory. It supports our heart health by improving cholesterol levels and regulating blood pressure.

Salmon is also very rich in potassium – another ally for our blood pressure – and in vitamins D, B12, B3 and B6, so critical for our immune and nervous systems.

Most famously, salmon is a fantastic source of Omega 3 essential fatty acids, which are, as the name suggests, essential for the good functioning of our body.

They protect and promote heart and brain functions, they support the nervous system and they balance hormone production and activity. They also control inflammation and immune response.

Ginger and lemon are also superfoods, so helpful in supporting our gut health and immune system.

GOOD OLD FASHIONED CHICKEN SOUP

This traditional chicken soup is still an immune-boosting power house.

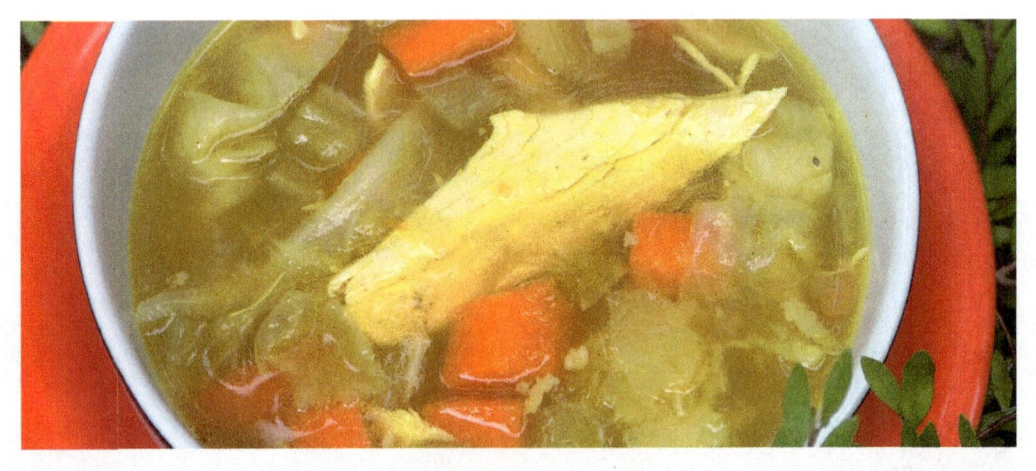

Ingredients

- 1 whole chicken (I recommend free-range, organic, hormone- and antibiotic-free)
- 1 green cabbage, cut into small chunks
- 1 large carrot, cubed
- 5 celery stalks, cut into 1-inch pieces
- 1 big white onion, diced
- 2 two-inch pieces of ginger, diced
- 1 head of garlic, separated into whole cloves, skins removed
- Salt & pepper

Directions

1. Rub the chicken with salt inside and outside to clean it. Rinse well and pat dry.
2. Gently salt the inside for seasoning. Use 1/2 teaspoon or less, depending on size of chicken.
3. Put onion and garlic into a large soup pot with 8 cups of water.
4. Bring to a boil and add the chicken. Top up the water to cover the chicken if necessary. Boil gently for about 40 minutes. Chicken should start to fall off the bone. You can start to gently pull it apart with a spoon.
5. Add the rest of the ingredients to the pot, season with salt and pepper. Boil for about 20-30 minutes longer, or until carrot and celery are soft but not mushy, and onion is translucent.
6. Turn off the heat and skim fat off the top.
7. Pull chicken out, remove bones from the pot. Pull out any large pieces of meat, shred and return to pot. Remove any meat still on the bone, return to pot. Stir gently and serve.

Recipe contributed by: The Cancer Coach, www.thecancercoach.org

OVEN-BAKED CHICKEN, BROCCOLI AND MUSHROOMS

Easy and flavourful dish for the whole family.

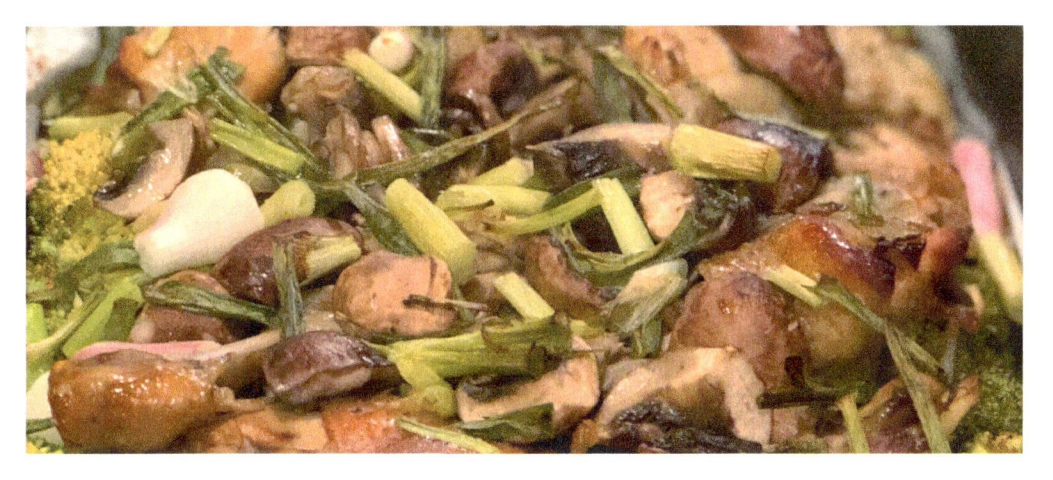

Ingredients

- 8 chicken legs
- Coconut aminos sauce
- 10 stems spring onion cut into 1-inch slices
- 1 bulb of garlic, whole cloves separated and peeled
- 1 big white onion cut cubed
- 250g whole mushrooms
- 1 broccoli crown separated into florets

Directions

1. Preheat oven to 180C.
2. Rinse and pat dry 8 chicken legs with thighs attached. Rub chicken with 1 tablespoon of olive oil or coconut aminos sauce.
3. Heat 2 tbsp. olive oil in a skillet. Add chicken and lightly pan-fry until golden brown. Set aside on a rack to drain.
4. Place the stems of spring onion cut into 1-inch slices, bulb of garlic, whole cloves separated and peeled, 1 big white onion cut into cubes, the mushrooms and broccoli into a large bowl and toss together with 1 teaspoon salt and a little olive oil.
5. Add the chicken and toss again gently.
6. Place everything on a large baking sheet with sides and put into oven for about 30 minutes or until veggies are tender and a little crispy.
7. Try smashing the softened garlic cloves into the chicken and veggies when you eat them.

Recipe contributed by: The Cancer Coach, www.thecancercoach.org

BEETROOT & PUMPKIN GOAT'S CHEESE TERRINE

Perfect as a side dish or a main course for your vegetarian menu, this Beetroot & Pumpkin Goat's Cheese Terrine is so delicious and easy to prepare.

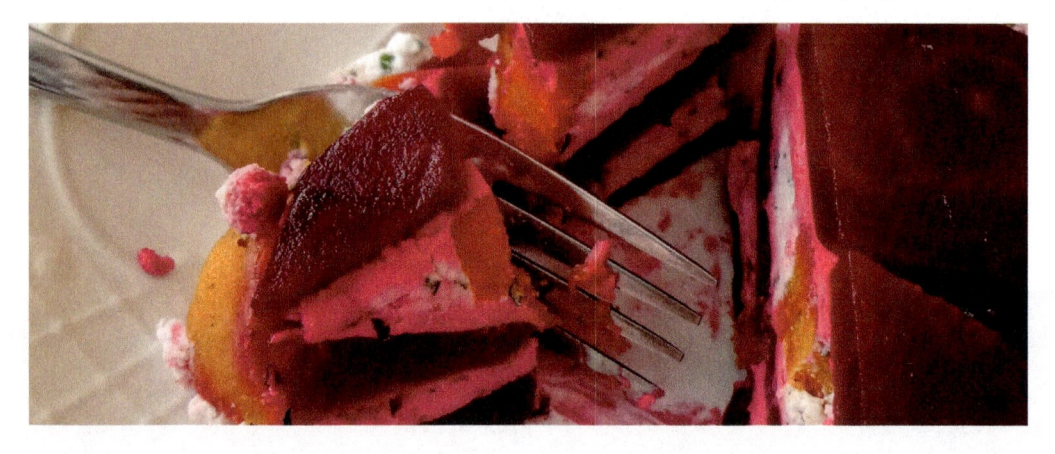

Ingredients

- 3 medium-large beetroot
- 1 miniature pumpkin or about 3 or 4 slices of a medium one
- 4 tbsp. freshly snipped chives
- 4 tbsp. freshly chopped parsley
- 1 tbsp. fresh or dried rosemary
- 1 tbsp. fresh or dried oregano
- 2 garlic cloves, finely chopped
- ½ tsp. freshly grated nutmeg
- 200g goat's cheese
- A pinch of good quality sea salt and black pepper

Directions

1. Line a 10 x 20cm loaf tin with baking paper, leaving enough paper to fold and cover the terrine later.

2. Scrub the beetroot and place them in a pot. Cover with water and lid, and cook for about 30 minutes until tender. Set aside to cool, then peel.

3. Peel and cut the pumpkin into small chunks, about 0.5-1 cm thick.

4. Put them in a pot with the grated nutmeg and half of the rosemary, and mix well.

5. Add some water, cover with a lid and cook for about 10-15 minutes, until tender. Set aside to cool.

6. While your vegetables are cooking, mix the goat's cheese with all the herbs and garlic in a bowl and season to taste.

7. Slice the cooked beetroot in various sizes, some about 0.5cm, some thinner.

8. Put a layer of beetroot on the bottom of the tin, followed by a thin layer of the goat's cheese and herbs mix.

Recipe contributed by: Silvia Mensurati, www.nutritiontoheal.com

9. Then, put a layer of pumpkin followed by another thin layer of the goat's cheese and herbs mix.

10. Repeat until you reach the top.

11. Cover the terrine with the baking paper, place a weight on top and refrigerate overnight or for 8 hours to set.

12. When ready to serve, cover the loaf tin with a plate and turn it upside down to remove the terrine.

Slice and enjoy!

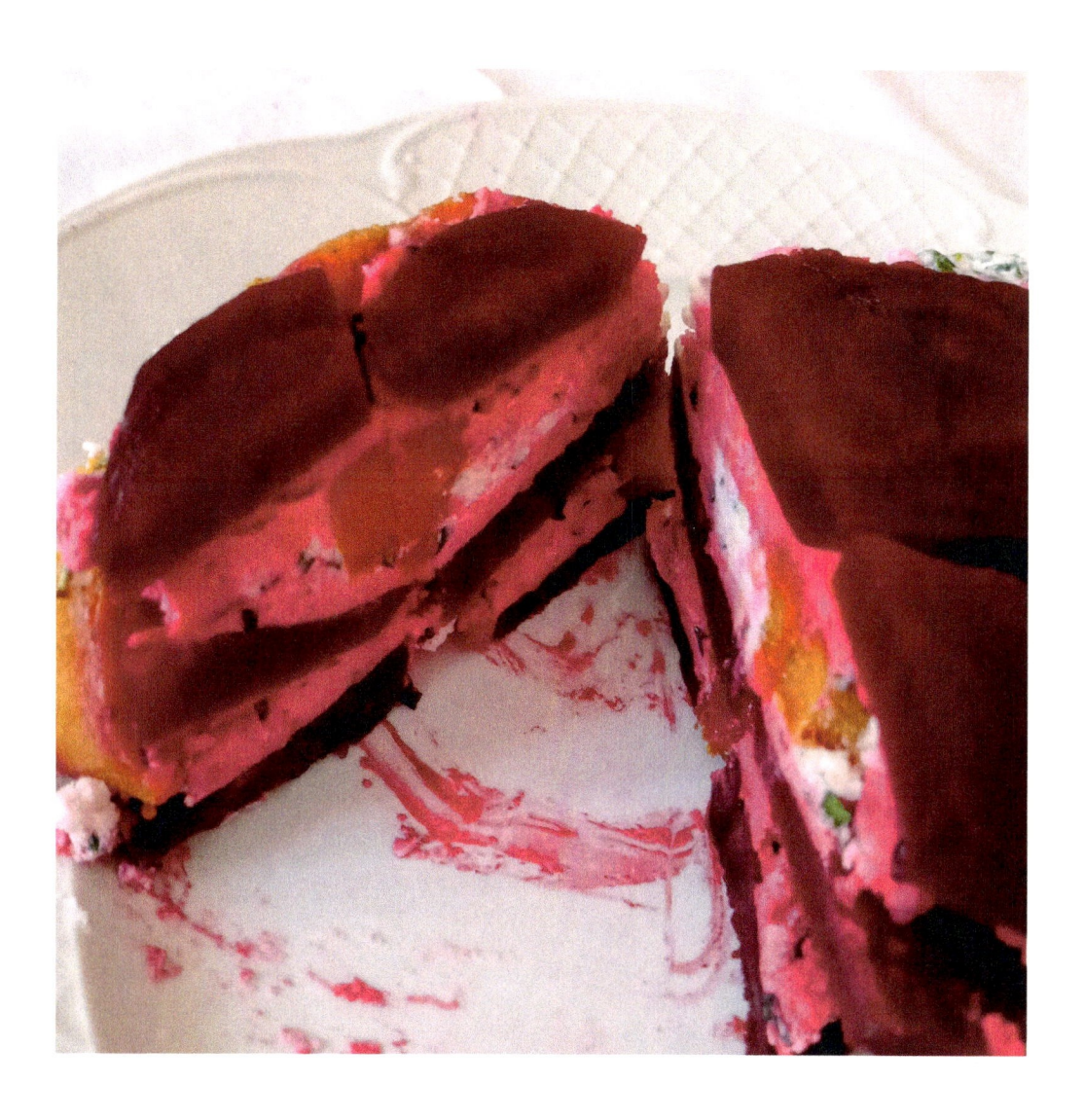

LAMB AND VEGETABLE CURRY

Easy and flavourful dish for the whole family.

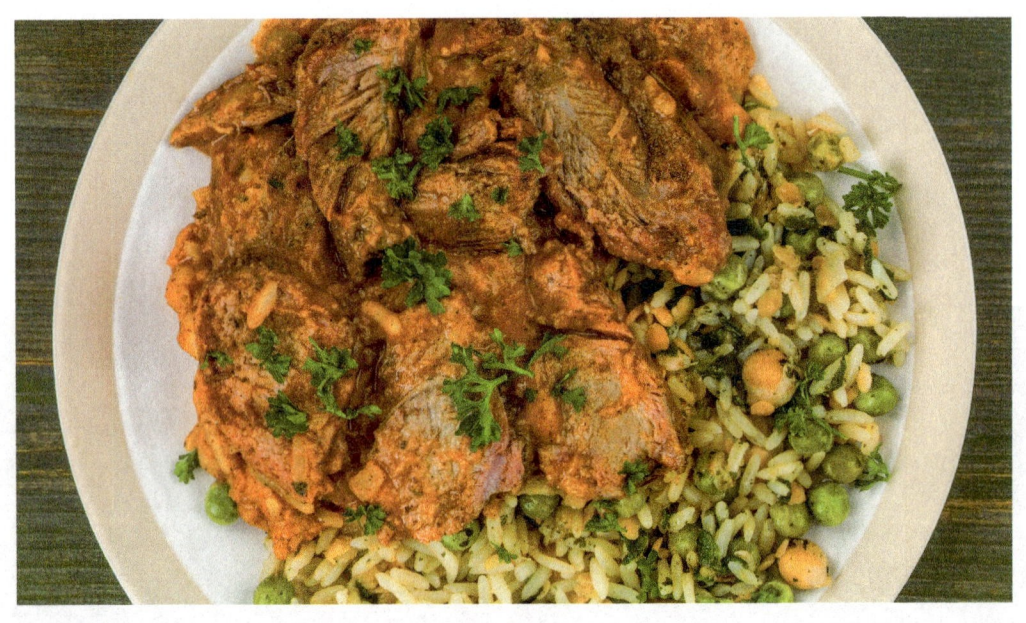

Ingredients

- 500g lamb (cubed)
- 1 tbsp. olive oil
- 1 tbsp. whole cumin
- 1 tsp. curry powder
- 1 red chilli, deseeded
- 2 medium onions, peeled and finely chopped
- 4 garlic cloves, peeled and finely chopped
- 2.5 cm piece root ginger, peeled and grated
- ½ cauliflower florets
- 2 large carrots, peeled and thickly sliced
- 2 tomatoes
- 300 ml broth
- 1 pak choi (chopped)

Directions

1. Using a frying pan with a lid, gently heat the olive oil, add the cumin until the seeds pop, then add the lamb.

2. Cook until brown, then add the onions, garlic and ginger and cook, stirring frequently, for around 10 minutes or until the onion is tender.

3. Add the curry powder, cauliflower and carrots and stir to mix well. Add the tomatoes and broth and bring to the boil. Reduce the heat to a simmer.

4. Cover and cook for around 1 hour until the lamb is tender.

5. Add the chopped pak choi and cook for around five minutes.

6. Can be served on a bed of spiralised courgettes.

Recipe contributed by: Jenny Phillips, www.inspirednutrition.co.uk

SATAY NOODLES

Easy and flavourful dish for the whole family.

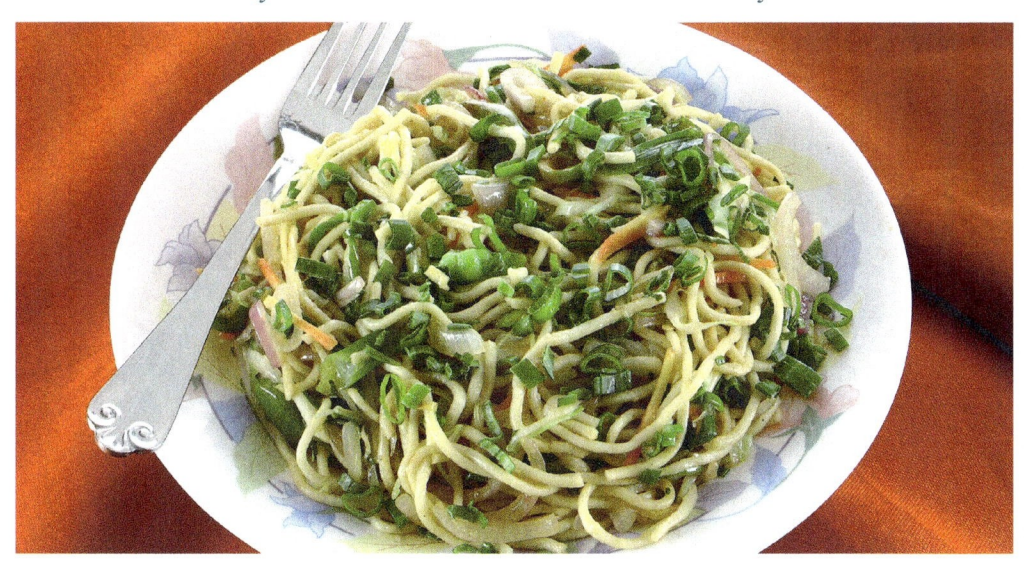

Ingredients

- 1 large courgette
- 1 sliced yellow pepper
- 100g mangetout, steamed
- 100g of mixed bean sprouts (e.g.: aduki, lentil, chick pea, mung)
- 1 tbsp. sesame seeds
- 2 tbsp. tamari
- 120g almond butter
- 2 tbsp. melted coconut oil
- Squeeze of lemon
- Pinch of chilli flakes

Directions

1. Spiralise the courgette to make noodles (or use a julienne knife or mandolin)

2. Place the noodles, pepper, mangetout, bean sprouts and sesame seeds in a bowl. Mix well.

3. Whizz together the dressing ingredients and pour over the vegetables. Mix well and serve

Recipe contributed by: Jenny Phillips, www.inspirednutrition.co.uk

STAR FISH PIE

Full of energy, full of flavour. An absolutely irresistible recipe!

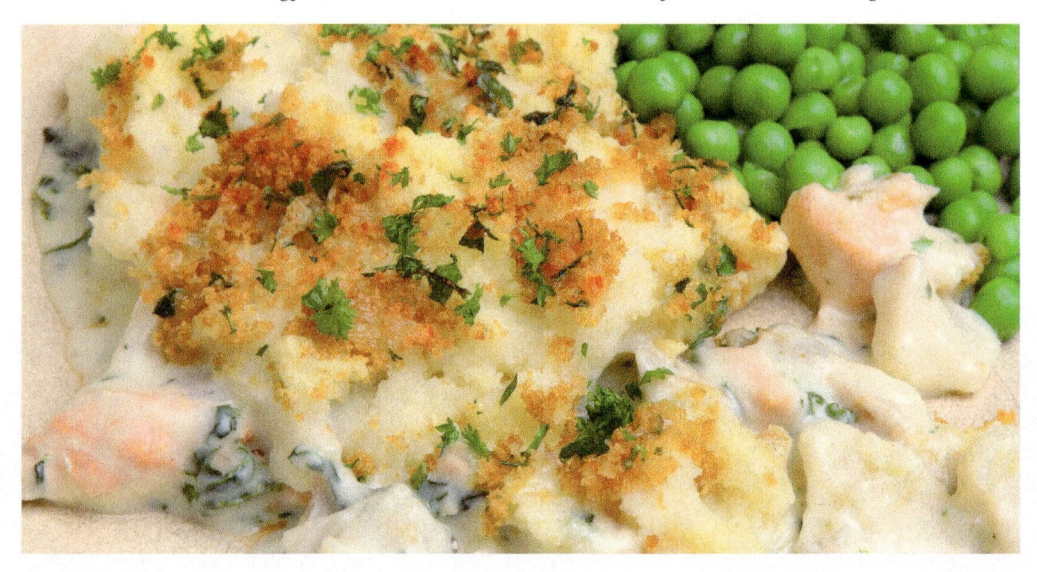

Ingredients

- 1 kg sweet potatoes
- 1 celeriac
- 1 carrot, chopped or spiralised
- 1 stick celery, chopped
- 200g coconut milk
- 1 red onion, chopped
- 2 cloves garlic
- 1 fresh red chilli
- 600g fish pie mix, haddock, cod and salmon

Directions

1. Peel and chop sweet potatoes and celeriac, place in a pan of water and boil for 20 minutes.

2. Sauté the onion and garlic for 2 minutes, then add celery, carrot, chilli, cook for another 2 minutes

3. Add the fish, then add the coconut milk.

4. Season with salt and pepper, add the parsley and then transfer the mixture into your ovenproof dish.

5. Once the sweet potatoes and celeriac are cooked, mash together and smooth over the fish.

6. Place in the oven at 200°C for 20 minutes.

7. Serve with a green salad.

Recipe contributed by: Jenny Phillips, www.inspirednutrition.co.uk

GRAM WRAP WITH HUMMUS, SESAME & LEMONY CARROT

Easy and flavourful dish for the whole family.

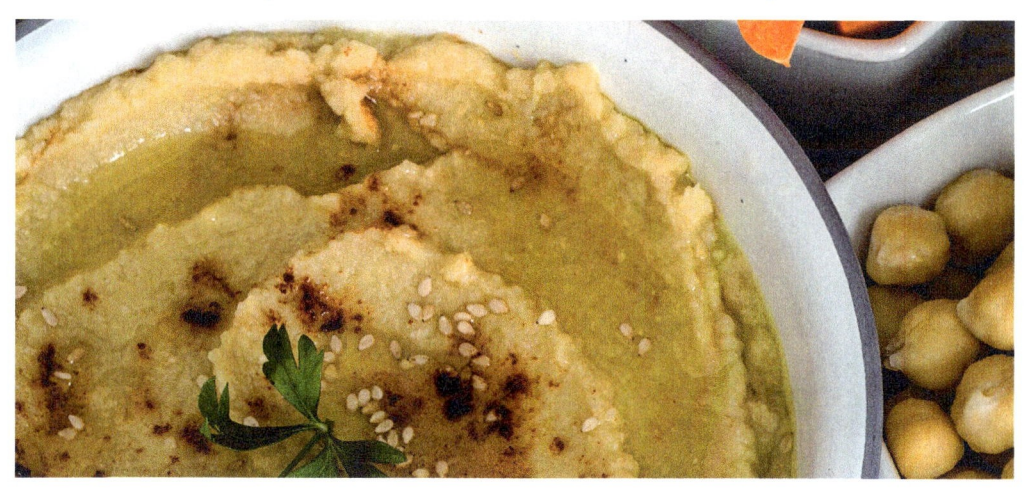

Ingredients

For the wrap

- 200g gram flour
- ½ tsp. cayenne pepper
- Salt
- ½ tbsp. turmeric powder
- 500ml water

For the filling

- 2 medium carrots (grated)
- Sesame seeds
- Zest of one lemon
- Olive oil or goose fat

Directions

1. Place the flour in a bowl add the cayenne pepper, salt and turmeric powder.
2. Make a hole in the middle and add the water.
3. Mix until blended.
4. Put some oil in a pan, you can use olive oil or goose fat.
5. Add one ladle of the mixture to the frying pan ensure it covers the bottom and gentle fry until golden brown. Place to one side keep warm.
6. To make the filling, grate the carrots and combine with the lemon zest, sesame seeds and a drizzle of olive oil.

Recipe contributed by: Jenny Phillips, www.inspirednutrition.co.uk

SIMPLE HEALING QUINOA

A few almighty herbs and spices are the highlights of this dish, chosen for their immune-boosting benefits.

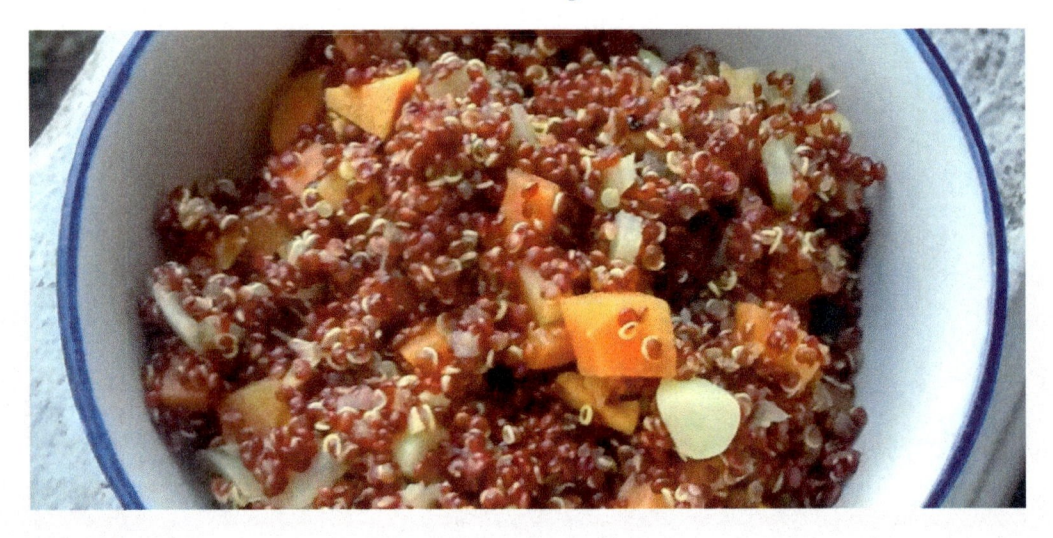

Ingredients

- 1 cup of organic red quinoa
- 5-10 garlic cloves, finely chopped
- 1 onion, finely chopped
- 1 carrot
- A good chunk of ginger, thinly sliced
- ½ tsp. of red chilli flakes or cayenne pepper
- 1 tsp. organic cold pressed coconut oil
- 2 cups of vegetable broth or water

Directions

1. Melt the coconut oil in a pan over low heat, add the onion and red chilli flakes and gently stir for a few minutes.

2. Add garlic and ginger and keep stirring for a minute or so.

3. Add the quinoa and carrot, stir for few seconds, and add the broth/water.

4. Cover the pan with a lid and bring to the boil.

5. Gently simmer for 10-15 minutes, until the quinoa has absorbed all the liquid and is ready.

6. You can also sprinkle some freshly chopped cilantro on top.

Recipe contributed by: Silvia Mensurati, www.nutritiontoheal.com

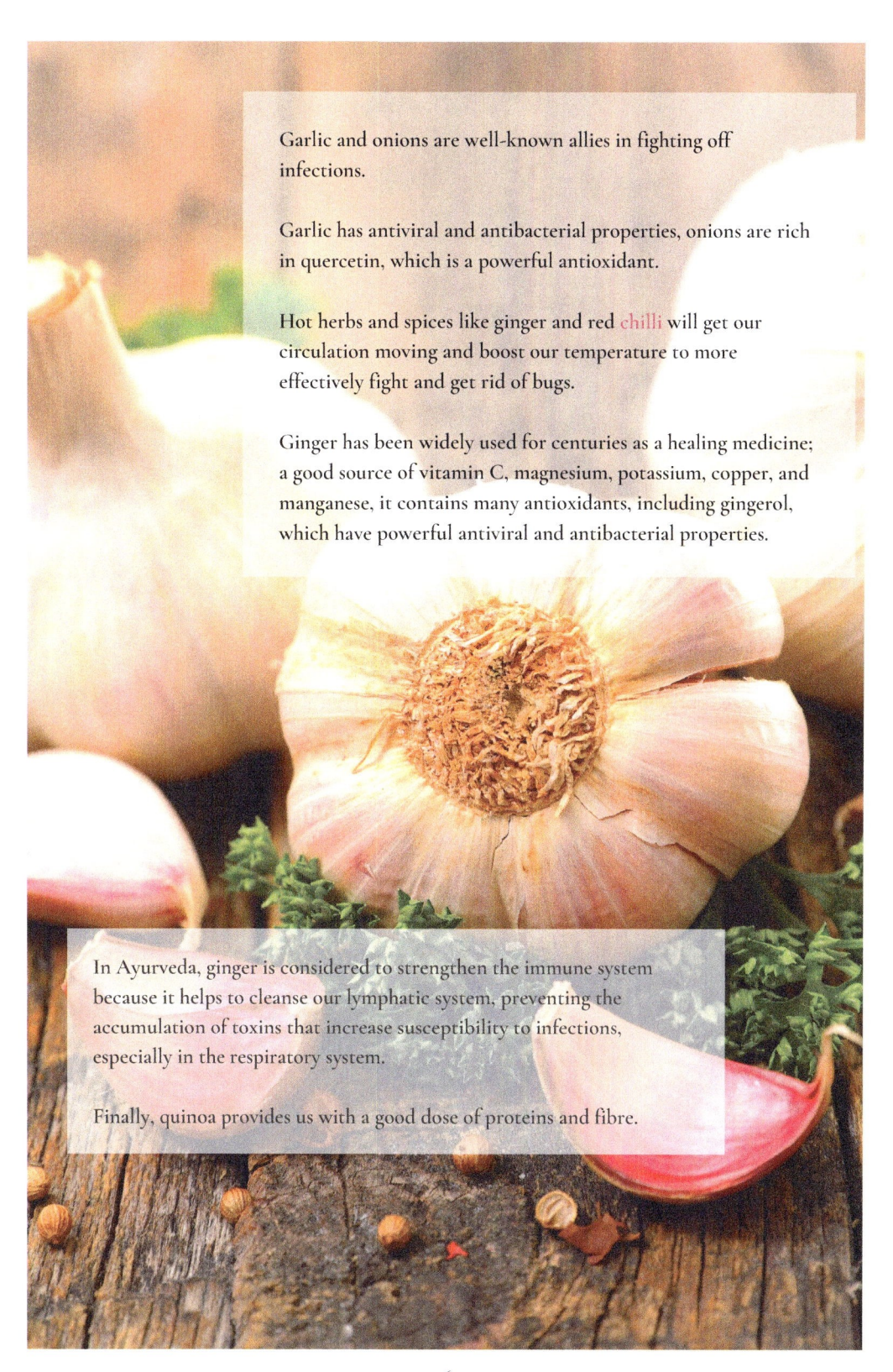

Garlic and onions are well-known allies in fighting off infections.

Garlic has antiviral and antibacterial properties, onions are rich in quercetin, which is a powerful antioxidant.

Hot herbs and spices like ginger and red chilli will get our circulation moving and boost our temperature to more effectively fight and get rid of bugs.

Ginger has been widely used for centuries as a healing medicine; a good source of vitamin C, magnesium, potassium, copper, and manganese, it contains many antioxidants, including gingerol, which have powerful antiviral and antibacterial properties.

In Ayurveda, ginger is considered to strengthen the immune system because it helps to cleanse our lymphatic system, preventing the accumulation of toxins that increase susceptibility to infections, especially in the respiratory system.

Finally, quinoa provides us with a good dose of proteins and fibre.

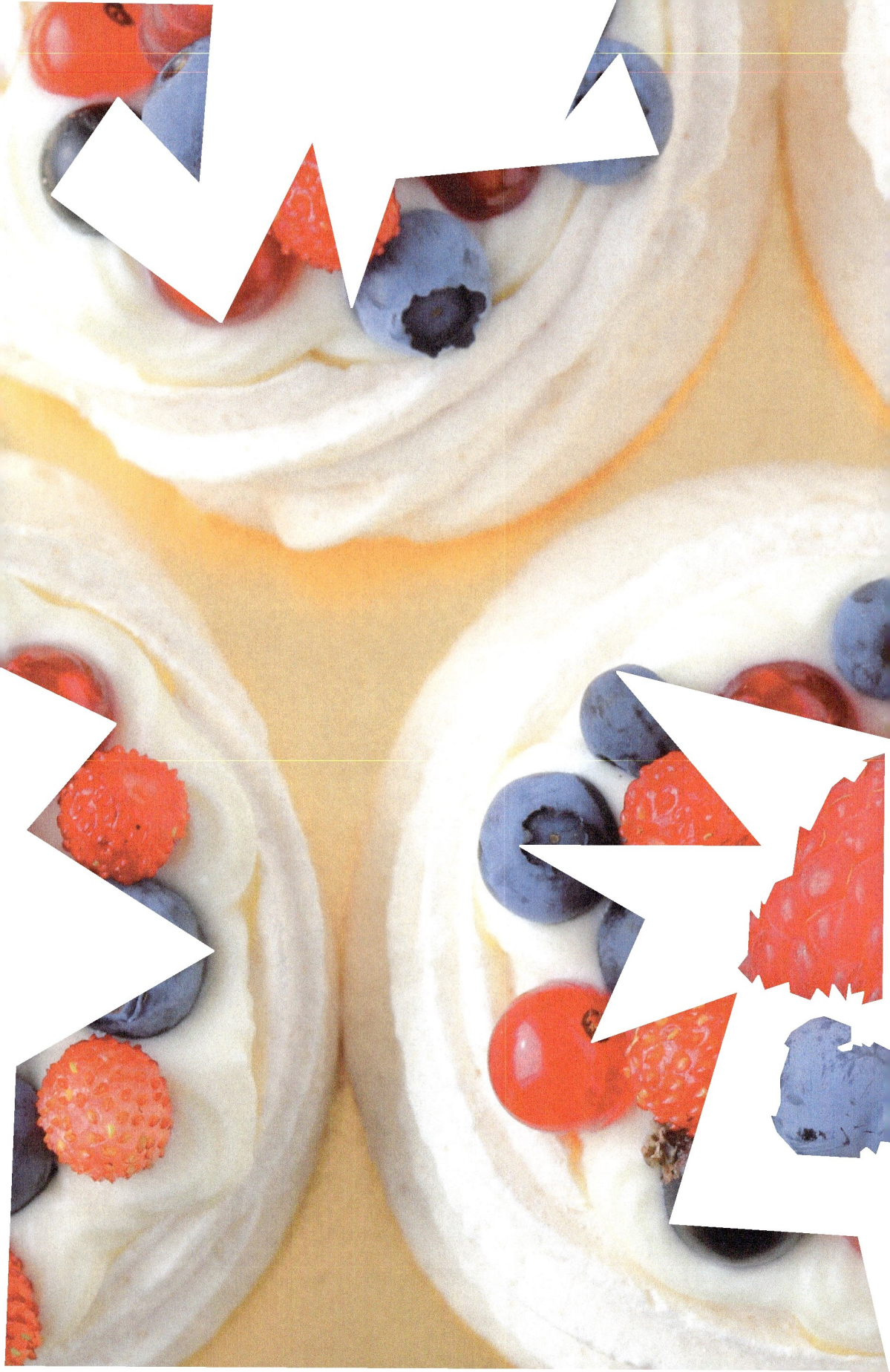

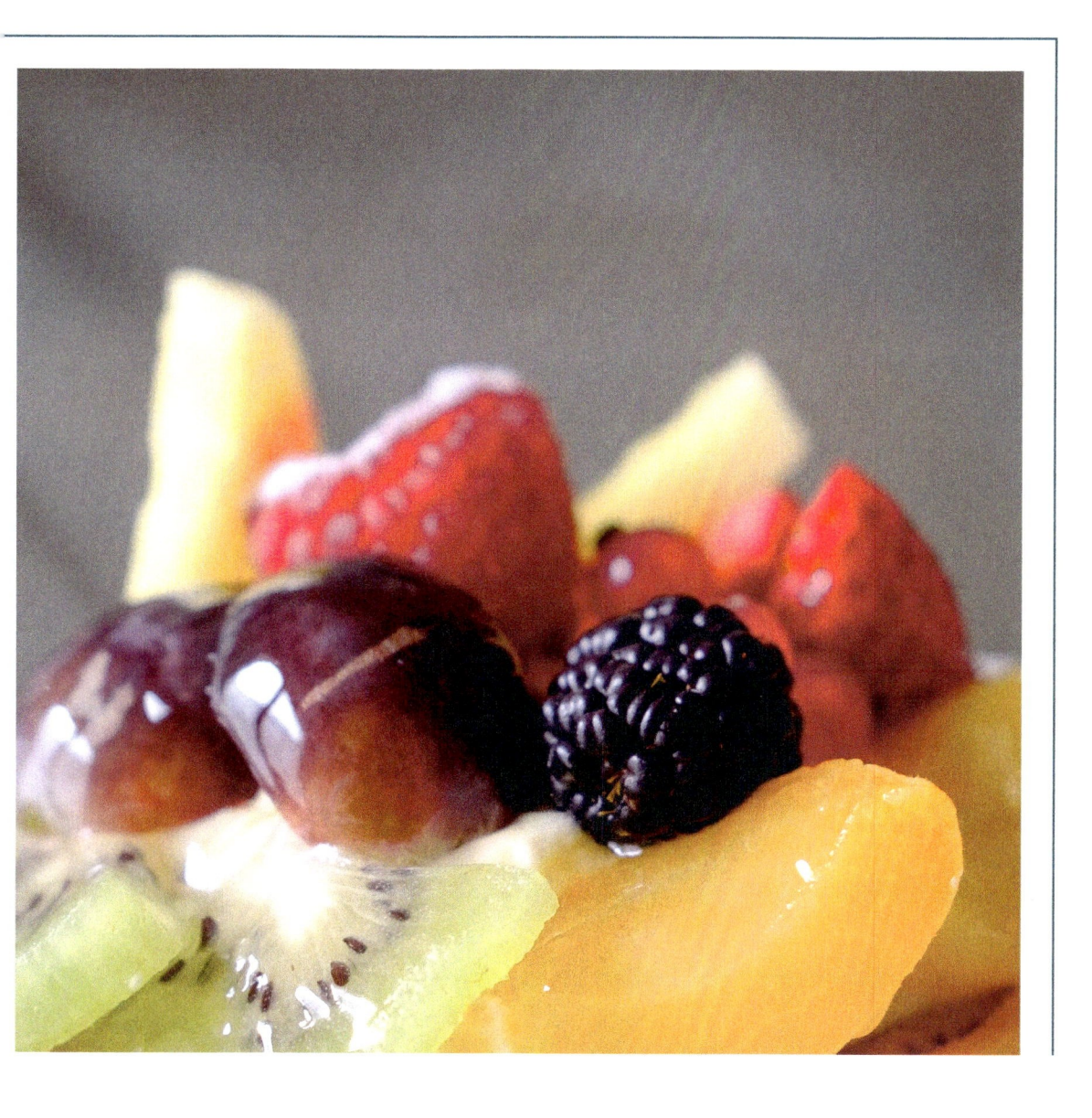

DESSERTS

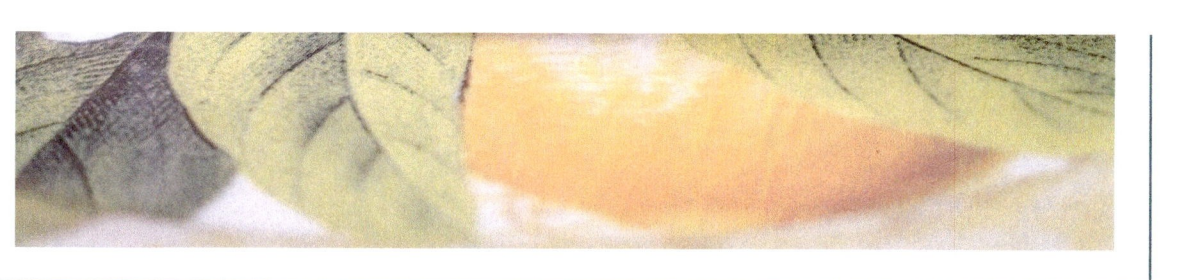

CHOCOLATE CHIA PORRIDGE

The love of chocolate with the power of chia. The perfect combination for an enjoyable dessert.

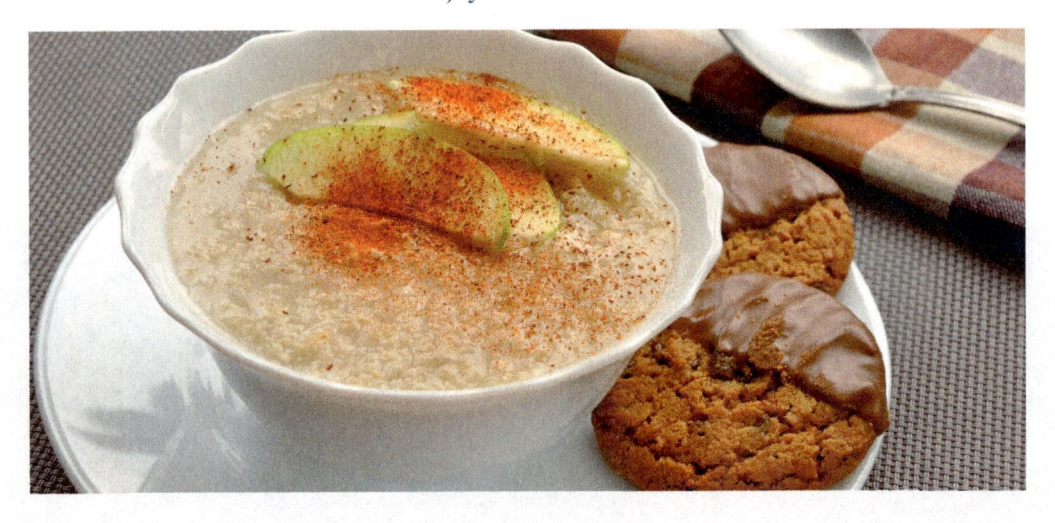

Ingredients

- 20g chia seeds
- Handful of almonds – soak in water overnight
- 1 cup warm water
- 1 apple
- 1 tsp. raw cacao (or organic cocoa powder)
- Pinch of cinnamon and 1 tsp. of flaked coconut (optional)

Directions

1. Core and chop the apple (skin on) - steam for 5 minutes.
2. Drain and rinse the almonds, add to a blender with water, apple and cacao and blitz.
3. Adjust to a thick but runny consistency by adding more water if required.
4. Pour over the chia seeds, stir well and leave for 10 minutes or overnight.
5. Sprinkle with cinnamon and top with coconut flakes.

Recipe contributed by: Jenny Phillips, www.inspirednutrition.co.uk

SENSATIONAL STRAWBERRY SMOOTHIE

This easy recipe brings the strawberry flavours to life!

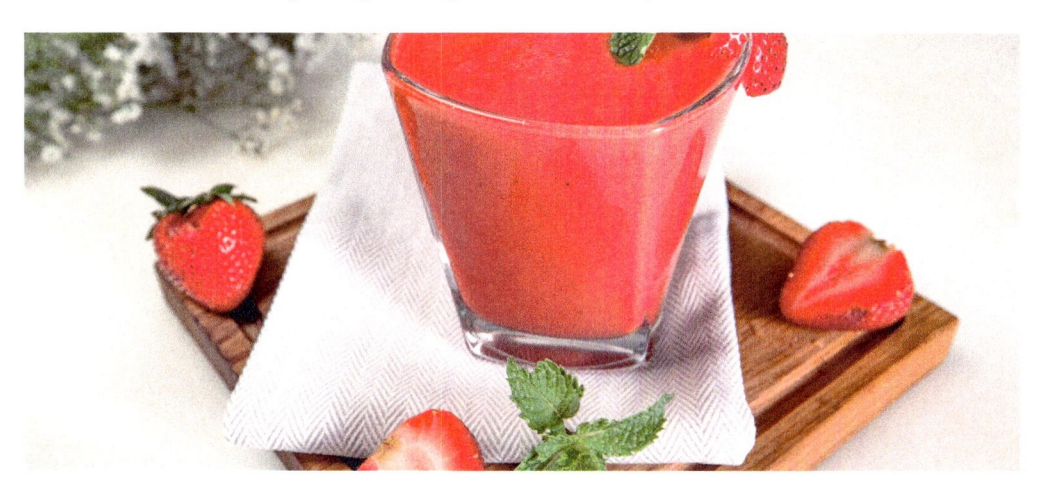

Ingredients

- Small handful of almonds, soaked overnight and drained
- ½ banana
- Handful of strawberries
- 1 tsp lecithin (optional)

Directions

1. Rinse the soaked almonds and place in blender with 200ml fresh water
2. Blitz and then use a nut milk bag to separate the sediment (this can be used in baking, freeze until ready to use)
3. Return the nut milk to the blender with banana, fruit and lecithin (if using)
4. Blitz and serve over ice

Recipe contributed by: Jenny Phillips, www.inspirednutrition.co.uk

BAKED PEACHES & COCONUT CREAM

For coconout lovers

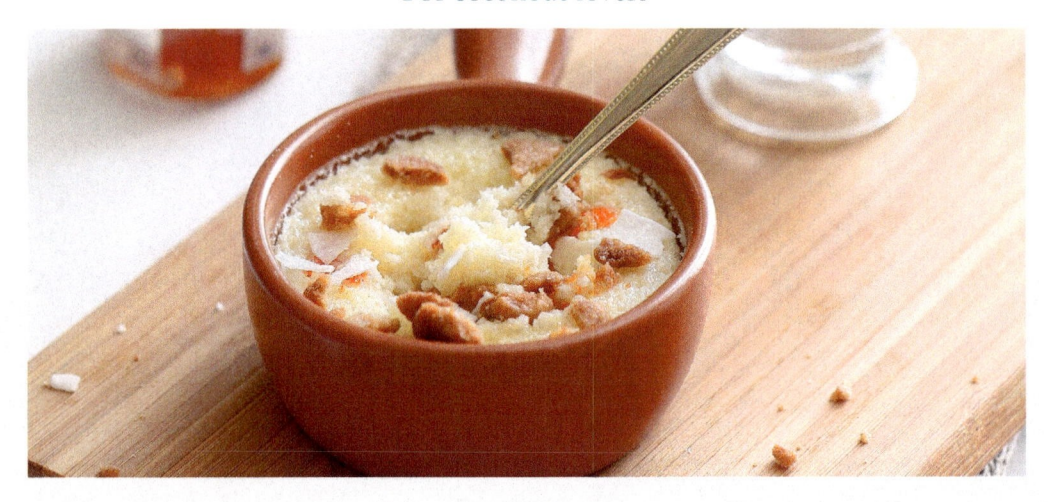

Ingredients

- 4 peaches, halved and pitted
- 50g of butter
- 30g coconut sugar
- 100g chopped mixed nuts
- Coconut cream to serve
- 1 tsp. honey (optional)

Directions

1. Melt the butter in a pan, stir in the sugar and then mix in the nuts

2. Spoon into the peach halves. Place in an ovenproof dish, cut surface uppermost

3. Bake in a hot oven – 190°C - for 15 minutes

4. To make the coconut cream: refrigerate a tin of coconut cream for 24 hours.

5. Scoop out the heavy cream, add the honey (if using) and whip until light and creamy.

Recipe contributed by: Jenny Phillips, www.inspirednutrition.co.uk

VEGAN-FRIENDLY MANGO ICE CREAM

This is fabulous, quick and vegan-friendly.

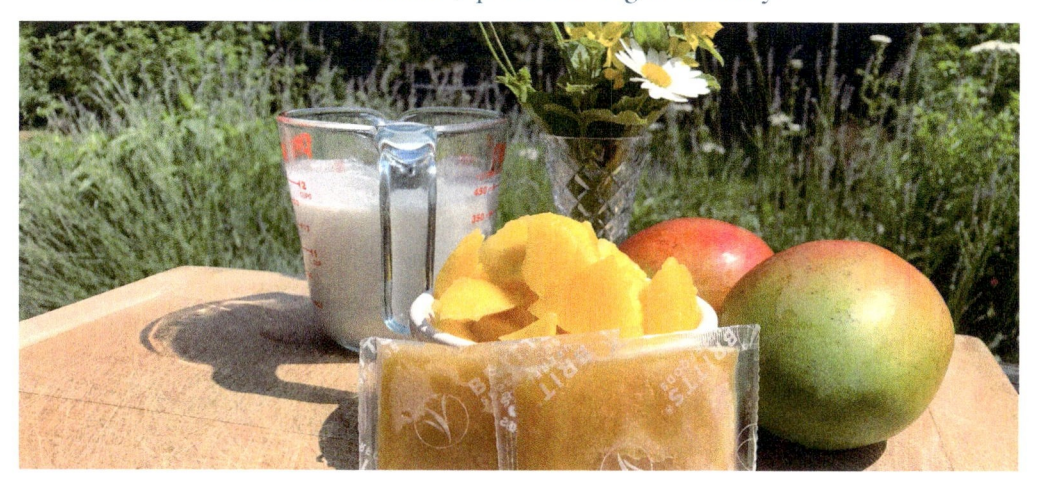

Ingredients

- A can of coconut milk
- 2 mangoes
- 2 sachets of Britt's Superfoods Ginger
- Turmeric juice

Directions

1. Simply chop the mangoes and mix all ingredients together in a blender. If you have one, add to an ice cream maker, if not, pour into a container and freeze.

2. Remember to stir every hour or so.

3. The finished product is simple and fabulous.

Recipe contributed by: Dr Britt Cordi, www.brittsuperfoods.com

HOMEMADE GRAPE SORBET

Frozen grapes on their own are a refreshing treat in hot weather. Blending them with a little honey and lemon, makes a sublime dessert.

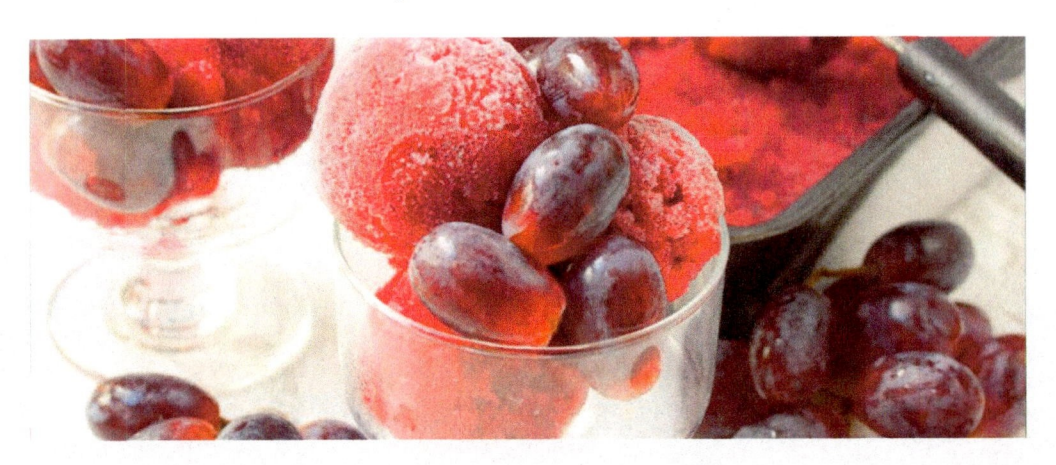

Ingredients

- 1 bunch seedless red or green grapes
- 1 tsp. honey
- 1 tsp. lemon zest
- 1 tsp. lemon juice

Directions

1. Remove one bunch of seedless grapes from their stems.
2. Wash and gently pat dry. Place grapes on a baking sheet or plate and freeze in a single layer until firm, a few hours or overnight.
3. Purée the frozen grapes in a food processor or blender, scraping down sides.
4. Add honey, zest and juice. Purée a little longer until smooth.
5. Enjoy immediately or refreeze in small containers for a terrific anytime treat!

Tip: You can make sorbet with all different types of frozen fruit. Try using mango, pineapple, papaya, berries...or even a mixture of a few types.

Recipe from Food for Life series, Yes to Life

LUXURY CHOCOLATE BROWNIES

This delicious recipe is easy to make, gluten-free and packed with protein from ground almonds and eggs. There is natural sweetness from the banana and this is supplemented with xylitol, a sugar alcohol that doesn't affect blood glucose levels. A little bit of what you fancy can indeed do you good.

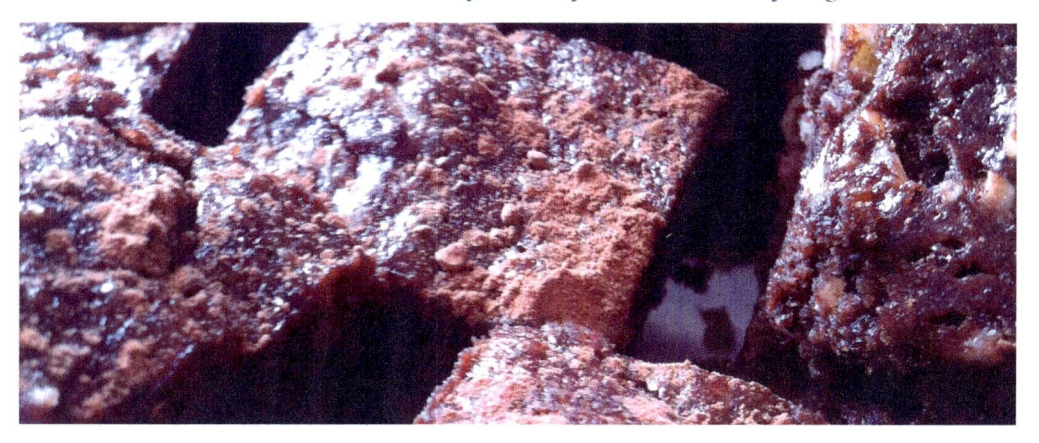

Ingredients

- 150g coconut oil or butter
- 90g honey
- 125g 70% chocolate
- 2 ripe bananas
- 2 tsp. vanilla extract
- 4 eggs
- 2 tsp. baking powder
- 30g cocoa powder
- 150g ground almonds
- 200g walnuts, chopped.

One 9 inch square cake tin, lined.

Directions

1. Pre-heat the oven to 180°C.
2. Cream the oil and sugar together using a wooden spoon or mixer.
3. Break the chocolate into a bowl and melt by placing it over a pan of boiling water or place it in a steamer for a few minutes.
4. Mash the bananas with the vanilla extract. Beat the eggs in a bowl.
5. Mix the dry ingredients in a large bowl- almonds, baking powder, cocoa and walnuts.
6. Add each of the wet to the dry ingredients, stir to combine well.
7. Pour into the lined cake tin and bake for 20- 25 mins or until spongy to the touch.
8. Cool and cut into squares before serving.

Recipe contributed by: Jenny Phillips, www.inspirednutrition.co.uk

LOW CARB VEGAN CHOCOLATE GANACHE TART

This is a healthy recipe because it contains antioxidant-rich ingredients which are protective for people with cancer.

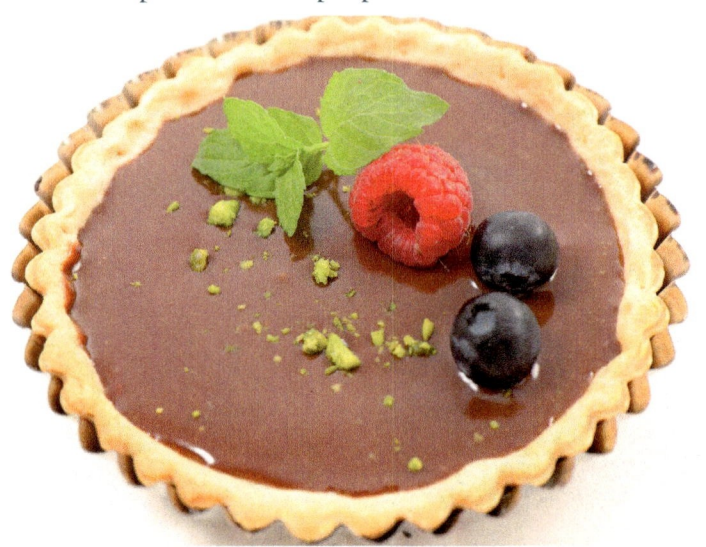

Ingredients

Crust

- 350 ml (170 g) almond flour
- 120 ml (45 g) cocoa powder
- 80 ml (70 g) erythritol
- 6 tbsp. coconut oil, melted

Filling

- 230 g (400 ml) dairy-free sugar-free dark chocolate
- 170 g coconut cream

Directions

For the Crust

1. Preheat the oven to 350°F (175°C).
2. Grease a fluted 9.5-inch (24 cm) tart pan.
3. Place the dry crust ingredients in a mixing bowl.
4. Add the coconut oil to the dry ingredients and mix well until completely combined.
5. Spoon the mixture into the pan and use your fingertips to press the base into place. Continue working until the base is evenly covering the base and sides of the pan.
6. Bake for 12 minutes. Remove and let cool while you prepare the filling.

Recipe contributed by: Gillian Bertram

7. To make the filling

8. Chop the chocolate into small pieces and place in a heatproof bowl.

9. Heat the coconut cream in a small saucepan, over medium-low heat until it is hot, but not boiling, whisking occasionally.

10. Remove the coconut cream from the heat and pour over the chocolate.

11. Let the mixture sit without touching it for two minutes.

12. Using a whisk, stir the ganache until it is smooth and glossy.

13. Let cool slightly before pouring into the tart shell.

14. Place the tart in the fridge to set.

15. Decorate by dusting with cacao powder and/or nibs.

I used 100% dark chocolate, the whole family loved it. I reduced the erythritol to one heaped teaspoon as I don't like things too sweet.

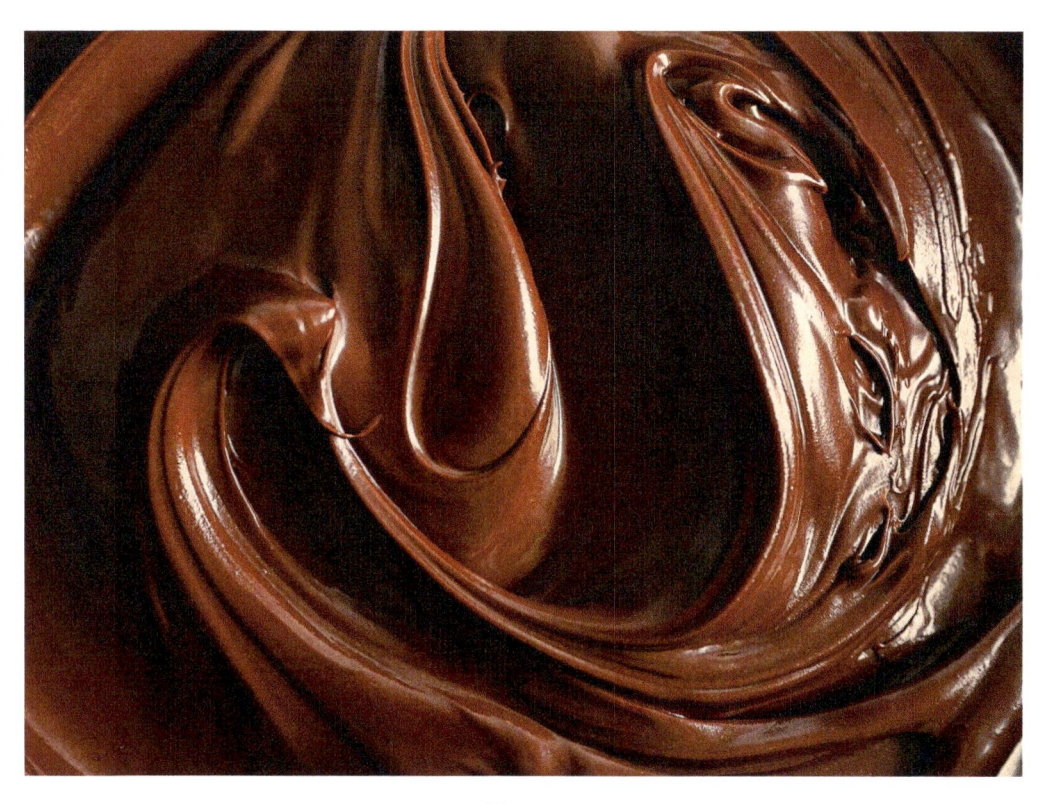

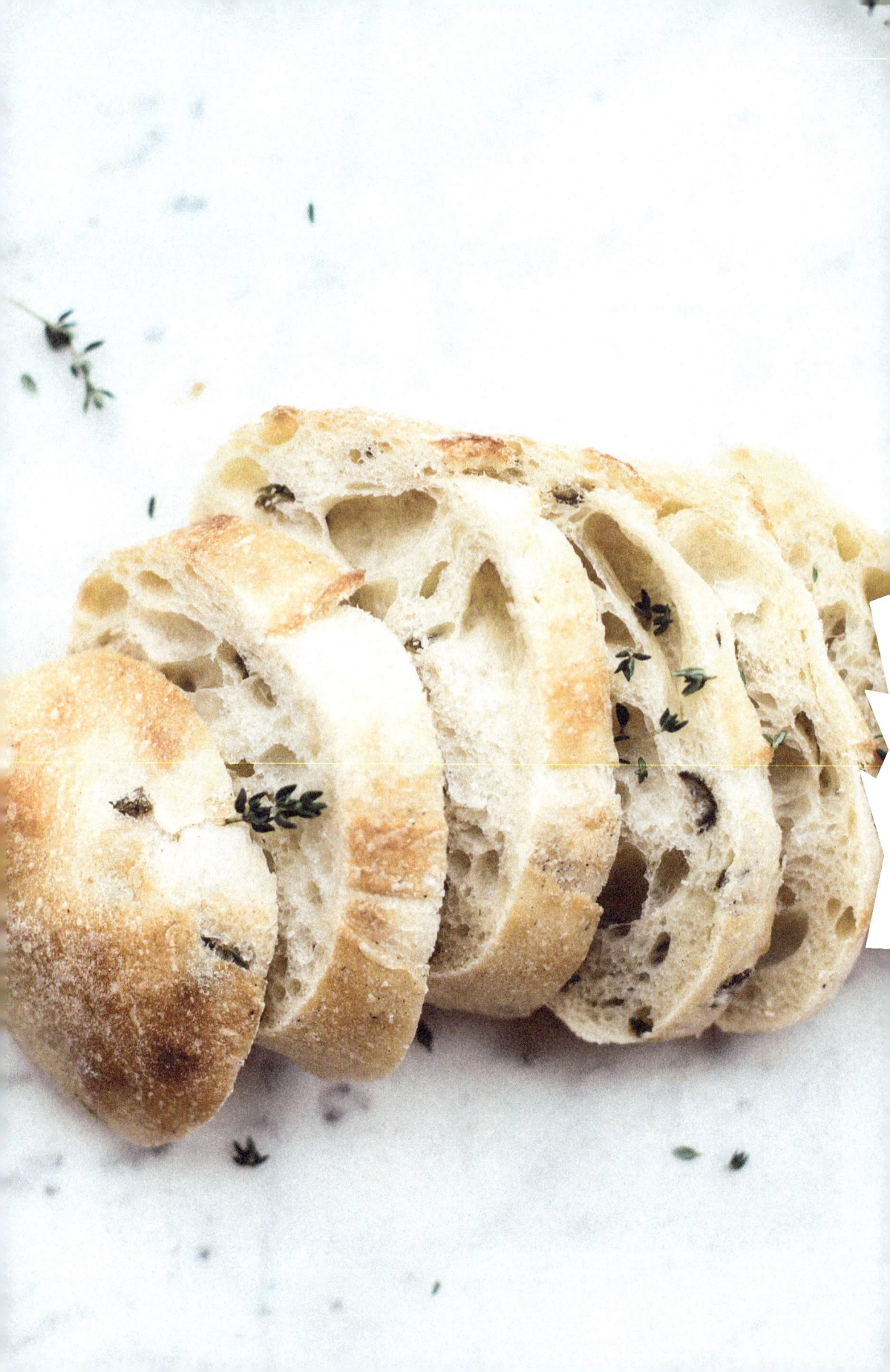

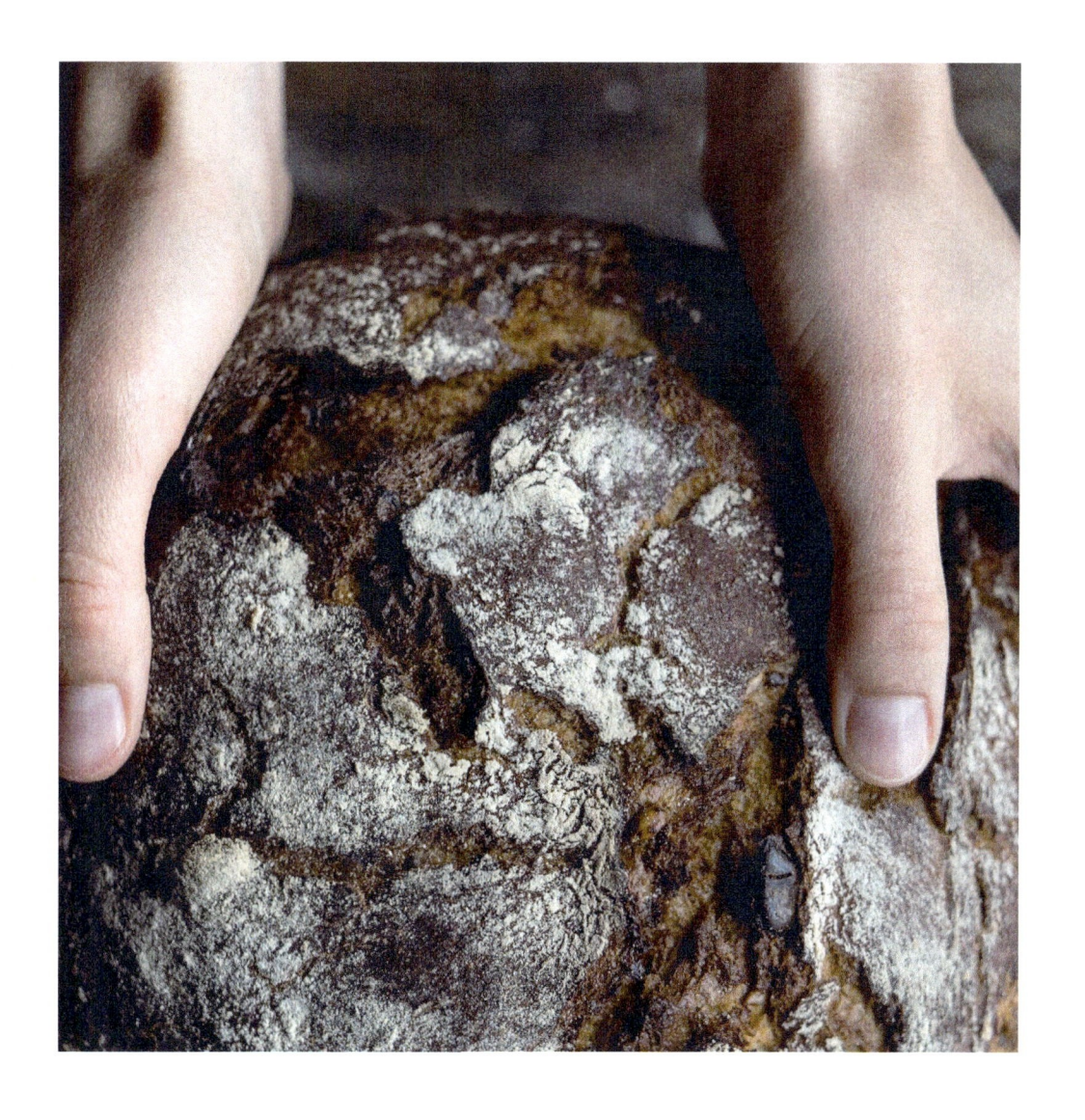

BREAD

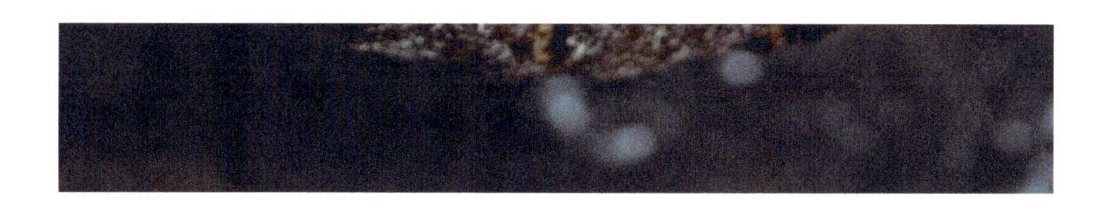

GLUTEN-FREE FERMENTED BUCKWHEAT BREAD

This is such a straightforward loaf in many ways - and I love that buckwheat flavour.

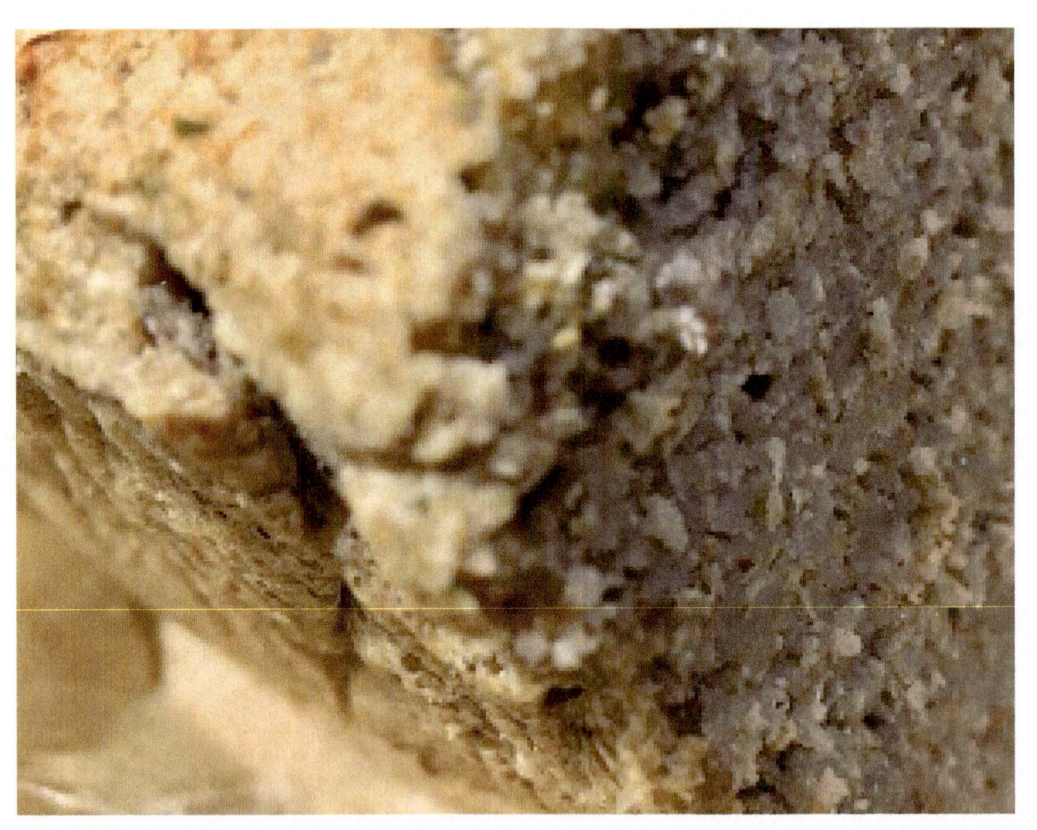

Ingredients

- 450 g buckwheat groats not toasted (2 1/2 cups)
- 3 cups of water for soaking the groats
- 330 g water for the batter (1 1/3 cups)
- 1/2 tsp. sea salt
- 1/3 cup pumpkin seeds
- 3 tbsp. of toasted flax seeds
- Several handfuls of pumpkin seeds and toasted flax seeds for decorating the top of loaf

Directions

1. Soak the buckwheat groats in water for 5-6 hours.

2. Drain the groats in a colander but do not rinse. The run-off will be very mucilaginous.

3. Blend the groats and new water in a blender or food processor. You may need to do this in two parts if you use a food processor, so as to not go over the top of the central blade tube and have leakage.

4. Pour into a glass bowl or large measuring Pyrex, and cover with a towel. This will be about 5 cups of batter.

5. Set aside for approximately 24 hrs at 67-70 F. Fermentation time is significantly shorter at warmer house temperatures or in the oven with the light on. Batter expansion is roughly from 5 to 6.5 cups. Do not mix the batter until the fermentation is finished or the batter will deflate, and it will be hard to calculate growth.

6. At the end of the fermentation, gently mix in the salt and any seeds you wish to add.

7. Pour the batter into the parchment paper-lined loaf pan, and decorate the top of the loaf.

8. Let the batter rise for another 30 minutes to an hour in your lit oven.

9. Preheat the oven to 350 F with pan in the oven.

10. Bake for approximately 80 minutes (less for a long narrow pan) or until the inside temp is about 200 F.

11. Remove from the oven and lift the parchment paper out of pan onto a cooling rack. Peel it off and let the loaf cool for at least 30 minutes before slicing.

Preparation time is around 30 minutes and cook time is around an hour and 20 minutes although we always seem to leave it a bit longer.

Enjoy!

Recipe contributed by: Philip Booth

THE LIFE-CHANGING LOAF OF BREAD

Great title for a loaf of bread!

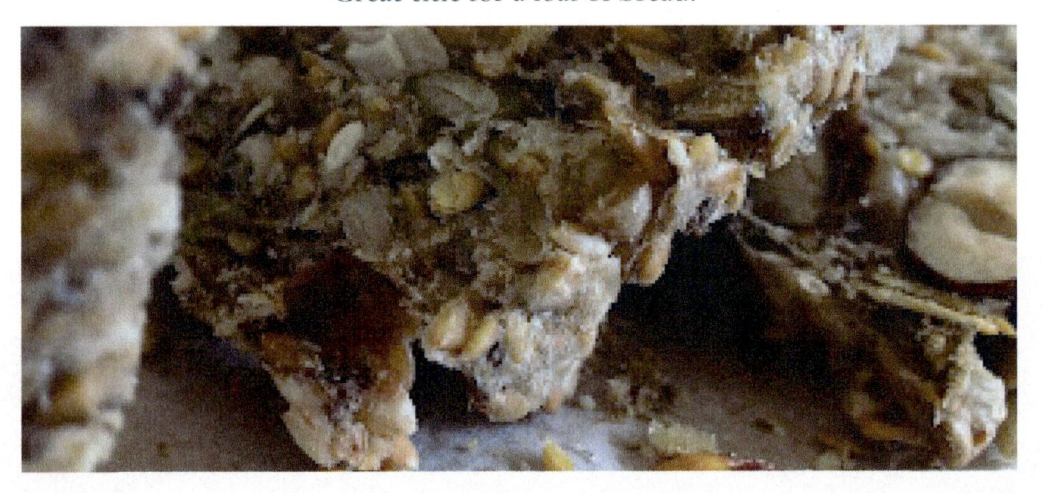

Ingredients

- 135g sunflower seeds and/or pumpkin seeds
- 90g flax seeds
- 65g hazelnuts or almonds (chopped)
- 145g rolled oats
- 2 tbsp. chia seeds
- 1 tsp. fine grain sea salt
- 1 tbsp. maple syrup (or alternatives like honey, pinch of stevia or your fancy)
- 3 tbsp. melted coconut oil or ghee
- 350ml water
- 4 tbsp. psyllium seed husks (3 tbsp. if using psyllium husk powder); this is the stuff that holds it all together so can't be missed out. It is hugely absorbent containing both soluble and insoluble fibre and soaking up ten times its weight in water. It can both sooth the digestive tract as well as helping remove toxins and can be used to reduce cholesterol levels, aid digestion, and alleviate both diarrhoea and constipation.

Directions

1. In a flexible, silicon loaf pan combine all dry ingredients, stirring well. You can use a bowl then an ordinary bread tin lined with parchment paper. This makes it so easy compared to all that 'mess' with flour - no kneading and no yeast or starter dough!

2. Whisk maple syrup, oil and water together in a measuring cup.

3. Add this to the dry ingredients and mix very well until everything is completely soaked and dough becomes very thick (if the dough is too thick to stir, add one or two teaspoons of water until the dough is manageable).

4. Smooth out the top with the back of a spoon.

5. Let sit out on the counter for at least 2 hours, or all day or overnight. To ensure the dough is ready, it should retain its shape even when you pull the sides of the loaf pan away from it.

6. Preheat oven to 175°C.

7. Place loaf pan in the oven on the middle rack, and bake for 20 minutes.

8. Remove bread from loaf pan, place it upside down directly on the rack and bake for another 30-40 minutes.

9. Bread is done when it sounds hollow when tapped. Let cool completely before slicing (difficult, but important).

10. Store bread in a tightly sealed container for up to five days. Freezes well too – slice before freezing for quick and easy toast!

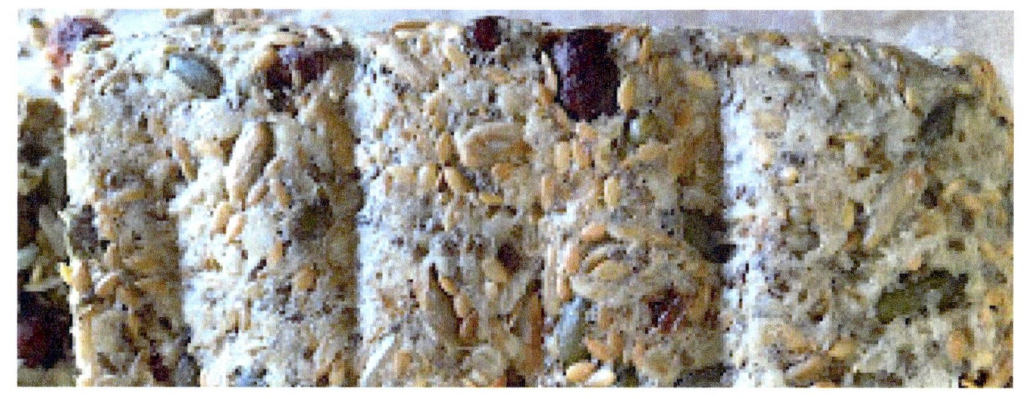

Recipe contributed by: Philip Booth

PECAN BREAD

Pecans are a good source of calcium, magnesium, and potassium, which help lower blood pressure.

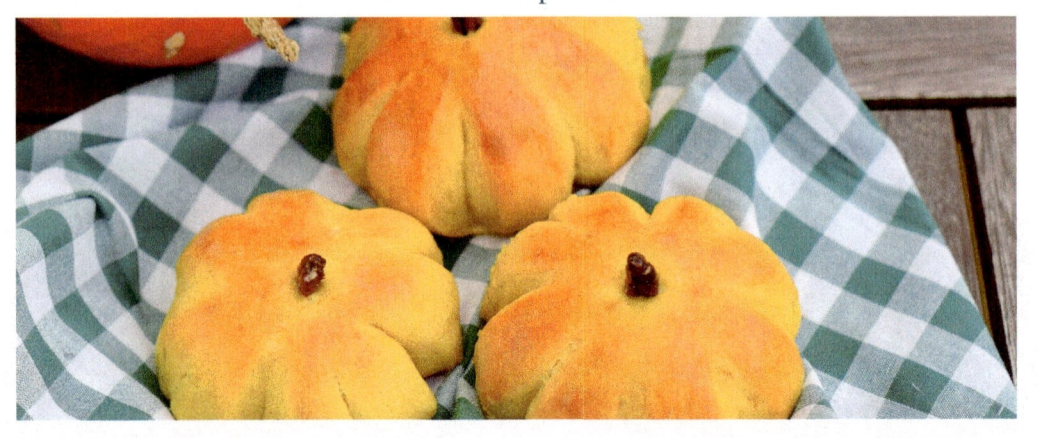

Ingredients

- 300g pecans
- 1 tsp. baking powder
- ¼ tsp. cinnamon
- 4 eggs
- 1 large ripe banana
- 2 tbsp. olive oil

Directions

1. Preheat oven to 180°C.
2. Grind the nuts in a blender.
3. Place in a bowl with the other dry ingredients.
4. Place the eggs, banana and oil in a blender. Blitz till smooth.
5. Pour the batter into the dry ingredients and mix well.
6. Spoon into a lined loaf pan.
7. Bake for 45 minutes.
8. Turn out and allow to cool.

Recipe contributed by: Jenny Phillips, www.inspirednutrition.co.uk

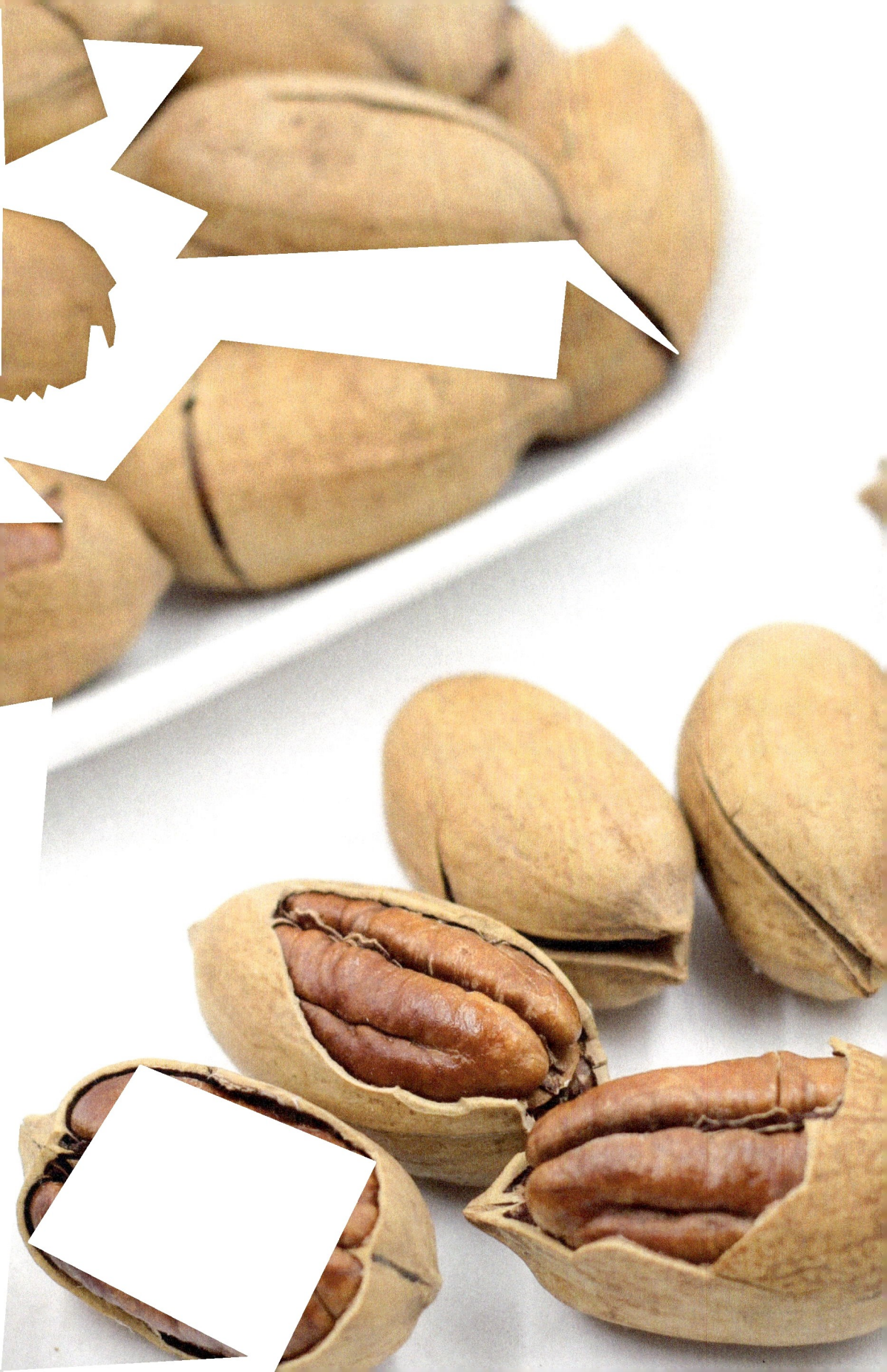

RECIPE INDEX

Tropical Bircher muesli	06
Omelette for mushroom lovers	07
Too good to be pancakes	08
Fruity chia porridge	09
Chia pudding	10
Cinnamon-spiced superseedy and apricot chewy flapjacks	11
Chia fresh summer pudding	12
Broccoli guacamole with poached egg	14
A taste of Tuscany on toast	15
Zesty fresh summer chia pudding	18
Beautiful beetroot dip	19.
Crunchy apple-cinnamon snack	20
Microwave hummus - from minimalist bakers	21
Flax & pumpkin turmeric thins	22
Buzz - worthy snack	24
Tamari seeds	25
Super-green smoothie	26
Healthy vegan crackers	27
Vegetarian easter energy eggs	28
Fresh greek salad (dairy-free)	30
Pea and lettuce soup	31
Prawn and blueberry salad with tangy avocado suace	32
Prawn and mango salad	34
A side of Vitamin C	35
All green quinoa salad	36
Simple stovetop veggies	38
Roasted butternut and pomegranate salad	39
Roasted cauliflower Indian style	40
Miso roasted mushrooms and spring onions with Japanese tamari superseeds	42

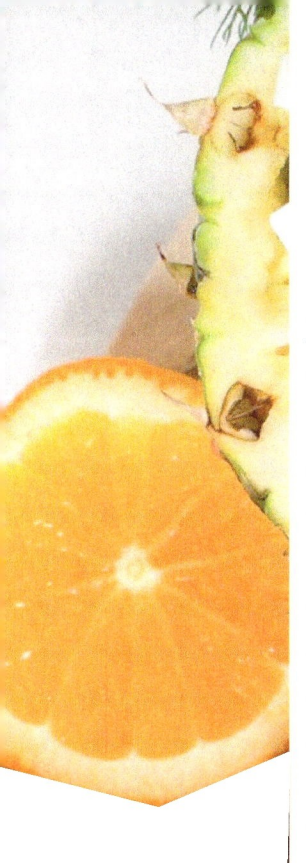

Jerk chicken salad	43
Kale and sweet potato chips	44
Tuna mix wraps	46
Mushroom soup	48
Vegan kale pesto	49
Asian baked fish parcels	50
Wild salmon in ginger lemon marinade	52
Good old-fashioned chicken soup	54
Oven-baked chicken, broccoli and mushrooms	55
Beetroot & pumpkin goat's cheese terrine	56
Lamb and vegetable curry	58
Satay noodles	59
Star fish pie	60
Gram wrap with hummus, sesame & lemony carrot	61
Simple healing quinoa	62
Chocolate chia porridge	66
Sensational strawberry smoothie	67
Baked peaches & coconut cream	68
Vegan friendly mango ice cream	69
Homemade grape sorbet	70
Luxury chocolate brownies	71
Low-carb vegan chocolate ganache	72
Gluten-free fermented buckwheat bread	76
The life-changing loaf of bread	78
Pecan bread	80

ABOUT YES TO LIFE

Yes to Life empowers people with cancer to make informed decisions about their cancer care options.

For 18 years, we have provided evidence-informed information to those in need.

Our aim is to provide information based on evidence to help people find out about Integrative Medicine, which we provide through a range of services.

Most importantly, we offer individual support through:

- our helpline
- our website
- information via blogs and publications
- our book, The Cancer Revolution
- the Yes to Life Radio Show on UK Health Radio
- the CancerTalk podcast
- workshops, talks and conferences
- our Wigwam Cancer Support Groups
- our Peer to Peer support service
- connecting people to a wide range of specialist therapies and practitioners

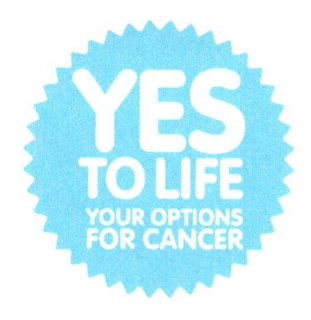

The UK's Integrative Cancer Care Charity

Yes to Life

Charity number 1112812
71-75 Shelton Street
Covent Garden
London WC2H 9JQ
Phone: 0203 222 0587
yestolife.org.uk
office@yestolife.org.uk

Helpline 0870 163 2990

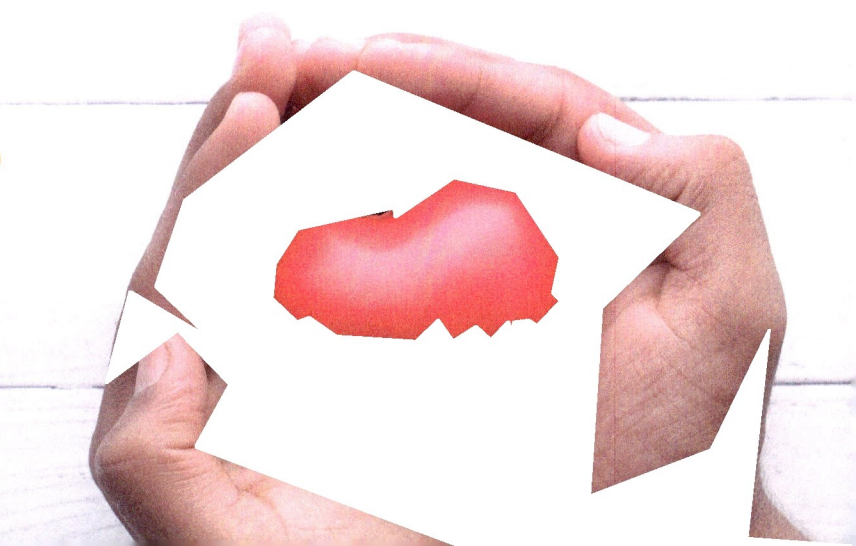

- @yestolifecharity
- @yestolife
- @yestolifecharity

Printed in Great Britain
by Amazon